Defend
your
Life

Defend *your* Life

A Safe, Easy, and Inexpensive Approach to Improving Quality of Life

SUSAN REX RYAN

Smilin Sue Publishing, LLC

DISCLAIMER

Published in April 2013 by Smilin Sue Publishing, LLC

www.smilinsuepubs.com

ISBN: 978-0-9845720-0-7

First Edition

Book design by Ambush Graphics

Edited by Jami Carpenter

Printed in the United States of America

Dedication

*To my wonderful husband Dave—who without question—
tirelessly loves and supports me. He is my world.*

Contents

Acknowledgments

Passion. Inspiration. Dedication. Commitment. Respect. Warmth. Understanding. Love. These words describe positive emotions of special people whom I wish to acknowledge.

First, I would like to thank Suzanne Somers for speaking "in plain English" about the value of pursuing natural solutions to health and aging issues. In 2007, I was seeking answers as to why I felt so poorly. Subsequently, I attended one of Suzanne's seminars and was captivated by her message. She helped me understand my issues and motivated me to address them to enjoy a better quality of life. Several years later I had the pleasure of meeting Suzanne after her lecture to members of the prestigious American Academy of Anti-Aging Medicine. I commended her for encouraging me to journey on the path to wellness. Thank you, Suzanne, for your tireless and impassioned dedication to promoting awareness of natural health and aging solutions to people from "all walks of life."

I extend my gratitude to those researchers, both scientists and medical professionals, who tirelessly conduct studies and trials to understand better vitamin D. I have been privileged to be in the same room with such renowned experts, including John J. Cannell, MD, Cedric F. Garland, DrPH, Frank C. Garland, PhD, Ed Gorham, MPH, PhD, William B. Grant, PhD, Robert Heaney, MD, and Reinhold Vieth, PhD. In addition, I offer the greatest respect and gratitude to other renowned researchers, including Edward Giovannucci, MD, ScD, Michael Holick, PhD, MD, Bruce Hollis, PhD, Joan Lappe, PhD, and Vin Tangpricha, MD, PhD.

Thank you to those who volunteer their valuable time to promote the wonders of vitamin D_3. Carole Baggerly is a breast cancer survivor who runs the non-profit organization Grassroots Health to educate medical professionals and the public about how vitamin D_3 may prevent cancer. John J. Cannell, MD, the founder and executive director of the Vitamin D Council, maintains an informative website about vitamin D and is a pioneer of "thinking outside the box" about the benefits of vitamin D_3.

Many thanks to Bobbie Christensen. Her sage tutelage from a seminar at the University of Nevada, Las Vegas has inspired me throughout the writing and publishing process.

Thanks to my friends who supported the effort to pen my first book. And, finally, my heartfelt thanks to my precious loved ones—my parents Janet and Robert Rex, my sister Cindy, her husband Guy, and the Ryan family—for their never-ending love and support. ☀

Introduction

An old adage suggests that everyone has at least "one book in them." I believe every human being on earth has at least one story to tell that could entertain, educate, or help people cope with life's challenges. An avid reader since elementary school, I dreamed of authoring a book, drafting title names, and musing about seeing my book in a library. Back then, there were neither chain bookstores nor the Internet. School libraries provided the primary source of my reading enjoyment, save the precious tomes that I owned.

My passion for reading and writing provides a vehicle to help others become aware of the marvelous benefits of vitamin D_3 supplementation. During vitamin D seminars in Toronto and California, the moderator challenged each participant to commit to how he or she would advocate the wonders of vitamin D_3. My response was to write a book that everyone could understand. Hence, here is my effort to promote understanding an easy, safe, and incredibly cheap solution to enjoying better health. Moreover, I sincerely hope that you will take action to make vitamin D_3 a routine part of your life and that others who are important to you will do so as well.

Defend Your Life comprises three parts. The first addresses the fundamentals of vitamin D_3 and its awesome benefits as well as minimal risk. The second highlights select diseases and conditions about which vitamin D_3 may offer protection.

The third includes my personal vitamin D_3 story, including my theory about adequate vitamin D_3 levels and how you can defend your life.

Reading this book will help you understand how adequate amounts of vitamin D_3 are essential to enhancing your quality of life. I endeavor to "spell out" how a simple, inexpensive, and safe solution—taking a daily vitamin D_3 drop or pill—may improve your life by minimizing the risk of contracting common contagious diseases as well as dreaded medical conditions, which include many types of cancer, heart disease, autism, and multiple sclerosis. ☀

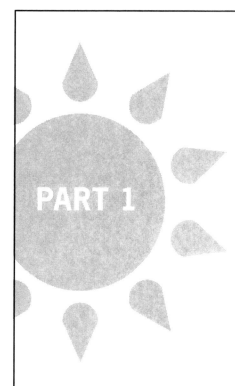

PART 1

Vitamin D Basics

Chapter 1

"Plane" Sense

Settling into my airplane seat, I felt relieved. I no longer needed to be concerned about packing, traffic, luggage, and airport security. Now I could relax! Looking forward to visiting my family in suburban Philadelphia, I briefly closed my eyes. But it was difficult to settle in completely as I knew someone would be occupying the seat next to me. Peeking into the seat pocket and finding a gently used, in-flight magazine, I tucked into a story that distracted me from the seemingly incessant line of boarding passengers, most of whom were concerned about stowing their carry-on baggage.

Near the conclusion of the boarding process, a slight, frail middle-aged man pointed to the unoccupied seat next to me. I stepped into the aisle, and he slowly slunk into the seat. Before fastening his seat belt, he donned a blue, surgical face mask. Sitting only a few inches from him, I could not help visualizing the then-recent media images of people in nearby Mexico wearing similar masks to attempt from spreading, or contracting, the highly contagious swine flu, or H1N1. The man coughed frequently into the mask and appeared to be in discomfort. He wearily rested his head against the seat back.

I glanced back and saw his wife sitting in the aisle seat directly behind me. Hmm … spouses usually try to change seats so they can sit together. Not this couple! A further glimpse around the aircraft revealed that the flight was completely full. Clearly there was nowhere to go. Suddenly my seat in a long metallic tube—soon to be airborne for hours—did not feel so comfortable. For a few minutes, I felt uneasy. Normally, I would worry during the entire flight about sitting inches from a person who possibly was suffering from a dreaded strain of a contagious influenza virus.

I was relaxed, however, knowing that my body most likely was protected, not only from my seatmate's germs, but also from the multitude of viruses and bacteria circulating throughout the aircraft. Why? I had discovered the wonders of vitamin D_3. I knew my body benefited from vitamin D_3 levels that protected my immune system from contagious infections and serious medical conditions such as heart disease, multiple sclerosis, diabetes, and some forms of cancer. Vitamin D_3 is defending my life, and most likely can provide the same benefits for you.

My name is Sue Ryan. I am neither a medical professional nor a celebrity. I am an American woman who suffered health issues for about a decade. Over the past several years, I have extensively researched vitamin D_3 to understand how its supplementation may improve the quality of my life. I intensively conducted my own research, earned continuing medical education units, and tenaciously monitored my vitamin D_3 levels. Thankfully, my health has significantly improved.

I marvel daily at the paramount role vitamin D_3 can play in our health. Adequate vitamin D_3 in the body possesses the potential to defend against a long list of diseases. Burgeoning medical studies have indicated that adequate levels of vitamin D_3 may prevent common and serious illnesses in the majority of the global population. Realizing the vast potential of improved quality of lives as well as millions of dollars saved by simply taking a daily, inexpensive supplement, I decided to write this book with the intent of providing easy-to-understand information that, if applied, may improve your health, lower your medical expenses, and enhance your quality of life. You can empower your health with vitamin D_3! ☀

Chapter 2

Vitamin D₃ Overview

Defend your gift of life. As human beings, we inherently possess an instinct for survival. We also, consciously or not, seek to improve our quality of the life we have been given. But the meaning of "quality of life" varies from person to person. If I asked 100 persons to define it, I probably would receive 100 different answers. I would surmise, however, that the majority of those responses would be related to good health. The state of being healthy, both mentally and physically, is a key factor to maintain or enhance one's quality of life. Our health affects virtually every aspect of our lives, from sleeping well to getting up each day and making a positive contribution to ourselves, family, friends, and employers. Yet our bodies are constantly subjected to millions of microbial invaders, attempting to challenge our immune system. So how do you defend your life? Ensure that your body enjoys adequate levels of vitamin D₃.

Sharing an interest in vitamins, a friend once asked me, "If you only could take one daily vitamin supplement, which one would you take?"

I replied, "Vitamin D_3."

Somewhat astonished, she clarified, "Vitamin D_3, not just vitamin D?"

I responded, "Not vitamin D or D_2, but vitamin D_3. Studies have indicated how beneficial vitamin D_3 is to our cellular and bone health, and the prevention of some cancers and other diseases, including multiple sclerosis. Here we are living in sunny Las Vegas yet many of us are deficient in vitamin D_3." I mentioned that my initial blood test results indicated that my vitamin D_3 levels were shockingly low. Consequently, I began taking daily vitamin D_3 supplements at a dosage recommended by my physician. In four months my vitamin D_3 levels increased significantly to a healthy range.

What is Vitamin D_3?

Vitamin D_3 is a steroid hormone, produced by our bodies when we:

a) Expose our skin to solar ultraviolet B (UVB) rays under optimal conditions;

b) Consume large quantities of fatty fish and vitamin D-fortified foods; or

c) Take vitamin D_3 supplements.

Unless you bask daily in UVB rays under optimal conditions, eat immense amounts of wild-caught, fatty fish, or take an adequate vitamin D_3 supplement, you probably have inadequate vitamin D_3 levels that may increase your risk of developing medical issues.

Why Do We Need Vitamin D₃?

Most Americans—across generations and geographical locations—suffer from deficient levels of vitamin D_3 because our lifestyle does not usually include vitamin D-rich foods or unprotected sunbathing. Recent medical studies indicate that low vitamin D_3 levels are associated with the increased risk of cancers including breast, colon, and prostate, as well as a host of other serious medical conditions, including heart disease, multiple sclerosis, autism, bone disease, and diabetes. Symptoms of low vitamin D_3 levels include common complaints such as muscle weakness, fatigue, and chronic back pain, as well as a susceptibility to contagious ailments such as the common cold. Vitamin D_3 deficiency is not only easy to diagnose by evaluating the results of a simple blood test, but can be readily resolved by taking inexpensive (not patentable), oral supplements.

What Are the Sources of Vitamin D₃?

Sunlight

As long as humans have roamed the earth, the sun has provided its light—including UVB rays—24 hours a day, 365 days a year. It is no coincidence that the most natural source of vitamin D_3 is exposure from the sun's UVB rays. People originally lived and worked outdoors. They wore little, if any, clothing. And they lived near the equator, the closest distance to the sun.

Fast forward to the Industrial Revolution in the nineteenth century, two twentieth-century world wars, vast technological advances, and global markets. Today people live and work indoors. They commute and travel by enclosed conveyances. Air conditioning has become widely used at work places and in homes. Food has become more and more processed, i.e., full of chemicals. Fast food was created. The list of actions and events that have contributed to the vitamin D_3 deficiency epidemic is long.

Let's briefly review a decades-old campaign launched by the cosmetic industry. Seeking additional revenue, the cosmetic industry endeavored to market its products as not only beauty but "health" aids. In the 1970s, the cosmetic business reportedly began funding medical schools' dermatology departments with the intent to influence the U.S. medical hallmark—the American Medical Association (AMA)—to warn the public about the dangers of sunlight. In 1989, the AMA issued the warning that caused millions to purchase and apply sunscreen and sunblock products. Well, you know the rest. The sun scare continues today. And so does the vitamin D_3 deficiency epidemic.

We do not need to hide our skin from the sun. The body possesses an inherent mechanism to produce just the right amount of vitamin D_3 from the sun. The skin can produce about 20,000 IU of "intake" vitamin D_3 a day depending upon a number of situational factors. After the body acquires enough D_3 (usually about twenty minutes of ideal UVB exposure), the skin's safety mechanism turns off the initial production of vitamin D_3. Moderate exposure to the sun is healthy.

A number of factors affect the degree of UVB sun rays absorbed by our bodies to produce vitamin D_3 including:

Geographic location. Your location is paramount to making vitamin D in your skin. The closer you are to the equator (lower latitudes) and the higher the altitude, the better your opportunity to acquire vitamin D_3-rich sunlight.

Time of day. The higher the sun is in the sky, the better to obtain vitamin D_3 from the sun. The hours of 10:00 AM to 2:00 PM are the best times to get vitamin D_3 from direct sunlight. If your shadow is shorter than your height, you are in a potential vitamin D_3-producing window.

Season. Many medical studies have demonstrated seasonal effects on vitamin D_3 levels. The sun shines the longest period of time during the summer and the shortest timeframe during the winter.

Cloud cover. An azure sky is highly preferable to cloud cover. UVB light is decreased by about 50 percent when penetrating cloud cover.

Air quality. An adverse product of industrial civilization is ozone pollution, which absorbs UVB sun rays before they can reach your skin.

Age. The older one is, the more challenging the effort to obtain and maintain adequate vitamin D_3 levels from sunlight. As people age, the concentration of the vitamin D_3 precursor (7-dehydrocholesterol) in the skin decreases.

Weight. Overweight and obese people have difficulty producing adequate vitamin D_3. As vitamin D_3 is fat-soluble, the body's fat cells absorb this essential nutrient, decreasing its availability to the organs, tissues, and cells.

Skin pigmentation. Melanin, the pigment in your skin, absorbs UVB rays. The darker your skin color, the more difficult it is to make vitamin D_3 in your skin. People with dark skin may require up to ten times the sun exposure that light-skinned people need to produce vitamin D_3. African Americans have staggering rates of low vitamin D_3 and accompanying incidences of medical conditions associated with vitamin D_3 deficiency.

Glass windows. Sunning by a glass window or door may feel soothing but it will not help you make vitamin D_3. Glass eliminates at least 95 per cent of UVB rays.

Sunscreen and cosmetics. The marriage of cosmetics and sun protection factors (SPF) will deny your skin the ability to make vitamin D_3. The application of either product to your skin most likely will block UVB sunlight.

Clothing. Not only are we encouraged to "cover up" in the sun but some clothing, including swimwear, contains SPF chemicals! The more clothing we wear in the sun, the less vitamin D_3 is produced in our skin.

Indoor UVB Light

As you learned, optimal conditions for producing vitamin D_3 from the sun are dependent on a number of elements. Some factors we can control, and others we cannot. So what about using indoor sources of UVB light to produce vitamin D_3 in our skin? For almost a century, UVB lamps have been used to treat medical conditions. Decades later, tanning beds became popular. People tend to frequent tanning facilities to look better, e.g., sport a tan during the winter. However, do they use tanning beds to increase their vitamin D_3 levels? They could under the correct circumstances. According to Dr. Michael Holick's 2010 book, *The Vitamin D Solution*, only one UVB lamp on the market was effective for producing vitamin D_3 in the skin.

Using indoor UVB light is an individual choice. Personally, I have not been inclined to utilize indoor tanning. I opt for outdoor UVB exposure and oral vitamin D_3 supplementation.

Food

Most American diets are not rich in fatty fish caught in the wild. Foods that naturally contain vitamin D_3 include salmon, mackerel, sardines, and cod liver oil (which contain a large amount of vitamin A, potentially causing vitamin A toxicity. See Chapter 5). In addition, a number of foods are enriched with "vitamin D" (either D_2 or the preferred D_3). Common vitamin D-fortified foods in the United States are milk, cereals, and fruit juices but they only contain small amounts of vitamin D. Enriched foods most likely will not effectively treat a vitamin D_3 deficiency because large quantities of these foods would need to be consumed daily. For example, you would need to drink ten 8-ounce glasses of vitamin D-fortified milk daily to obtain merely 1,000 IU of vitamin D.

Vitamin D₃ Supplements

The most practical and effective treatment of vitamin D_3 deficiency is to simply take a pill (soft gels are better absorbed) or liquid drop containing vitamin D_3, readily available online or in any drugstore, supermarket, or pharmacy without a prescription. As vitamin D_3 is fat-soluble, I believe the best time to take your supplement is during or immediately after your fattiest meal of the day.

How Do I Find Out My Vitamin D_3 Level?

The most accurate way to determine your vitamin D_3 level is to take a simple blood test from your healthcare practitioner. The name of the blood test is 25-hydroxyvitamin D or 25(OH) D. Owing to the medical findings over the past decade, routine blood work ordered by a practitioner often includes a vitamin D_3 evaluation. Nonetheless, double-check with your practitioner before your blood is drawn to ensure that the vitamin D_3 blood test is included on the laboratory order form. Many healthcare plans cover all, or at least partial, costs of the blood test. (The ICD-9 code is 268.9.) In addition, blood screening kits for 25(OH)D are available via online from reputable companies. See "Additional Resources" for some U.S. laboratories that perform 25(OH)D blood testing. My personal opinion is that a healthy range of circulating vitamin D_3 is at least a measurement of 50-80 Nano grams per milliliter of blood (ng/mL). See Chapter 18 for additional thoughts about optimal circulating vitamin D_3 levels.

Animals Also Need Vitamin D_3 for their Health

As you begin to understand the importance of vitamin D_3 to humans, are you wondering about other living creatures? All land vertebrates (animals with a backbone) require vitamin

D$_3$ for their health. Mammals, reptiles, and birds acquire the majority of their vitamin D$_3$ intake from casual exposure to UVB rays of sunlight.

What about your furry friends at home? Fur-bearing animals, including cats and dogs, need vitamin D$_3$, and naturally acquire the essential nutrient from sunlight. Although UVB rays cannot penetrate fur, animals consume cholecalciferol when they lick, or groom, their fur! Our cats Dima and Elizabeth were adamant about getting their daily sunshine. After sunning themselves, they luxuriously groomed their fur, demonstrating nature's way of ensuring that animals have sufficient vitamin D$_3$ to maintain their health.

Snakes, turtles, lizards, alligators, and other reptiles inherently sun themselves to warm their cold-blooded bodies and absorb UVB light to acquire their vitamin D$_3$ fix. Reptiles in captivity often suffer from vitamin D$_3$ deficiency. Young pet reptiles frequently have rickets, and older ones often endure osteoporosis.

Birds also indulge in sunning themselves to maintain their body temperature and to consume vitamin D$_3$. Similar to humans, birds sunbathe in a variety of positions, such as facing the sun with their feathers spread out for maximum exposure to UVB rays. By caring for their feathers, birds apply preening oil from the uropygial gland—located near the base of their tail—over their plumes to help the UVB light convert molecules in the oil to cholecalciferol, or vitamin D$_3$. Once again, nature dictates the magnitude of vitamin D$_3$ to living creatures.

Summary

Vitamin D_3 deficiency is easy to correct by increasing—ideally in concert with your healthcare practitioner—your intake of this essential nutrient. Sources of vitamin D_3 include UVB light, select foods, and supplements. In the next chapter I explain how vitamin D_3 works in the body. ☀

Chapter 3

How Vitamin D₃ Works

Let's look at how vitamin D₃ works in your body to protect you from developing diseases by understanding some basic medicine. Our health is controlled and maintained by trillions of cells, the smallest units in the human body. The body's organs comprise millions of cells and tissues. Cells contain components called receptors that control what vitamins, minerals, hormones, and other substances (medications, free radicals, etc.) can enter or depart a cell. The nucleus of every cell contains our genetic composition.

Vitamin D receptors (VDRs) receive and, in some cases, produce activated vitamin D₃. VDRs are present from head to toe: in our brains, eyes, hair, and skin as well as in our cardiovascular, endocrine, gastrointestinal, immune, musculoskeletal, nephrological, neurological, reproductive, and respiratory systems.

How is Vitamin D₃ Made in your Body?

The most natural way to obtain vitamin D₃ is from moderate exposure to ultraviolet B (UVB) rays from the sun. When your skin absorbs UVB rays, your body interfaces with a chemical called 7-dehydrocholesterol and produces initial vitamin D_3 (cholecalciferol). Adequate intake of vitamin D_3 supplements and foods also will result in the production of initial vitamin D_3.

Once initial vitamin D_3 is produced in our skin cells, it enters your blood stream and travels to the liver. The liver processes—by hydroxylation—initial vitamin D_3 into circulating vitamin D_3 (calcidiol or 25-hydroxyvitamin D). Circulating vitamin D_3 travels along two distinct paths. First, circulating vitamin D_3 is converted by your kidneys into activated vitamin D_3 (calcitriol or 1,25 hydroxyvitamin D). This activated vitamin D_3 interacts with your parathyroid glands to maintain calcium blood levels for strong bones and teeth. Second, if circulating vitamin D_3 remains in your bloodstream after calcium levels are maintained, the liver converts the leftover circulating vitamin D_3 into activated vitamin D_3. The "excess" activated vitamin D_3 travels in the blood to your tissues and cells and attaches to VDRs to perform functions essential to great health:

- Regulate gene expression.

- Reduce inflammation.

- Fight viral and bacterial infections.

- Regulate cell differentiation, proliferation, and natural death (apoptosis).

These mechanisms of action are vital to protecting you from developing a wide array of medical conditions including autoimmune disorders, cancer, heart disease, and influenza.

In addition, medical studies indicate that vitamin D_3's anti-inflammatory function may inhibit genetic aging.

How Safe is Vitamin D_3?

The primary purpose of this book is to highlight some of the amazing benefits of vitamin D_3 supplementation. But how safe is vitamin D_3 supplementation? The good news is that vitamin D_3 toxicity is rare.

As you have learned, vitamin D_3 supplementation mimics the production of cholecalciferol in your body when UVB rays strike your skin. Scientific studies indicate that our bodies can naturally absorb about 20,000 IUs from daily exposure to UVB sun rays to make a sufficient amount of vitamin D_3 to protect us from most illnesses. Thus, daily vitamin D_3 supplementation of about 10,000 IU probably is safe for most people. However, persons who suffer from kidney disease, sarcoidosis, or hyperparathyroidism should definitely consult a medical practitioner before taking vitamin D_3 supplements. In addition, folks who are using cardiac glycosides (digoxin) or thiazide diuretics should check with their healthcare provider prior to using supplemental vitamin D_3.

Summary

Too much vitamin D_3 in the human body is rare. Nonetheless, the safest method of controlling your vitamin D_3 supplementation is to monitor your circulating vitamin D levels at least every six months until you have achieved a vitamin D_3 status that works for you. ☀

Chapter 4

The Only "Real" Vitamin D

This book primarily addresses the importance of vitamin D_3's role in protecting your health and improving your quality of life. However, the fact that there exists a "third form" of vitamin D, i.e., vitamin D "three," begs the question, "What are the other types of vitamin D?" To the best of my knowledge, five forms of vitamin D have been identified by the scientific community. Here is a brief synopsis of each type:

Vitamin D_1: a molecular compound (1:1 ratio) of ergocalciferol and lumisterol.

Vitamin D_2: ergocalciferol or calciferol.

Vitamin D_3: cholecalciferol (The only "real" vitamin D!)

Vitamin D_4: dihydrotachysterol or 22,23 dihydroergocalciferol.

Vitamin D_5: sitocalciferol, produced from 7-dehydrositosterol.

Vitamin D_3 is the only "real" or bioidentical substance that supports the wide array of benefits stated in this book. Only UVB exposure, natural dietary products (certain fatty fish, etc.), and cholecalciferol (vitamin D_3) supplementation can ultimately initiate the vital communications with the vitamin D receptors in your cells, tissues, and organs to perform the plethora of positive functions to defend your life!

All other forms, or analogues, of vitamin D—including high doses of vitamin D_2 available only by prescription in the United States—are synthetic compounds that have been chemically altered. Taking these other vitamin D forms, in my opinion, is like attempting to fit a square peg into a round hole; the square peg simply does not fit. You would be wasting your time and money.

What about Vitamin D_2?

Although vitamins D_1, D_4, and D_5 are rarely explored in scientific literature, vitamin D_2, or ergocalciferol, remains a topic of discussion. Vitamin D_2 is derived from irradiated yeast or mushrooms and widely used in food and beverage fortification. High-dose (50,000 IU) vitamin D_2 is only available by prescription. However, lower dose vitamin D_2 is available over the counter. Vegans and some vegetarians have preferred to take vitamin D_2 supplements, since vitamin D_3, until recently, was an animal product made from lanolin in sheep's wool. Vegan vitamin D_3 supplements, made with lichen extract, have become widely available online.

For decades, the medical community presumed that both forms of vitamin D were equivalent, owing to studies of rickets prevention in infants. In the late twentieth century, realizing the importance of measuring circulating vitamin D to ascertain (and usually to improve) vitamin D levels in humans, researchers examined vitamin D_2's effectiveness in raising circulating vitamin D_3 levels.

How Does the Effectiveness of Vitamin D_2 and Vitamin D_3 Compare?

In 1998, Canadian scientists, including distinguished vitamin D expert Reinhold Vieth, conducted a study on humans to understand the perceived equivalence of the two useable forms of vitamin D. Their data indicated that vitamin D_3 increased humans' circulating vitamin D more efficiently than vitamin D_2. Furthermore, the study suggested the nutritional value of vitamin D_3 is probably greater than that of D_2.

Six years later, Creighton University researchers studied the potency of vitamins D_2 and D_3 by administering singles doses of 50,000 IU of these two forms of vitamin D to twenty healthy males. After tracking circulating vitamin D levels over twenty-eight consecutive days, the scientists surmised the potency of vitamin D_2 is less than 33 percent that of vitamin D_3.

According to a study published in the *American Journal of Clinical Nutrition* in 2006, Lisa Houghton and Reinhold Vieth concluded that vitamin D_2 should no longer be equivalent to vitamin D_3 for supplementation and fortification. The researchers based their conclusion on D_2's diminished usefulness in raising circulating vitamin D levels as well as the D_2's shorter shelf life.

Vitamin D expert Michael F. Holick, PhD, MD, offered opposing results of the effectiveness of vitamin D_2 versus D_3. According to the March 2008 report published in the *Journal of*

Clinical Endocrinology and Metabolism, Dr. Holick and colleagues disagree with previous reports that vitamin D_2 is less effective than vitamin D_3 in raising circulating vitamin D levels. During the 2007 winter and early spring, the researchers conducted a randomized, placebo-controlled, double-blinded study of 68 healthy humans, aged 18-84 years old, over an eleven-week period. Eighty-seven percent of the subjects began with circulating vitamin D levels less than 30 ng/mL, a measurement that most vitamin D experts now consider to be sub-optimal. The data collected during the study suggested that vitamin D_2 enjoys the same effectiveness as vitamin D_3 in maintaining circulating vitamin D levels.

Note: According to the report's Disclosure Statement, Dr. Holick serves on the Speakers' Bureau for pharmaceutical companies including "Merck, Proctor and Gamble, and Eli Lilly" and as "a consultant for Amgen, Novartis, Quest Diagnostics, Proctor and Gamble, and Merck." Richard Reitz, another scientist who was involved in the study, disclosed that he is the "Medical Director of Quest Diagnostics/Nichols Institute and has equity interests in Quest Diagnostics/Nichols Institute." The eight remaining researchers stated that they "have nothing to declare." In his 2010 book, *The Vitamin D Solution*, Holick summarizes the D_2 versus D_3 debate by stating that D_2 is "currently the only FDA-approved vitamin D available to physicians to treat and prevent vitamin D deficiency at this dosage, and it works well."

Vitamin D researcher Robert P. Heaney, MD, led a single-blind, randomized trial to compare the potencies of vitamin D_2

and vitamin D_3. Published in a 2011 edition of the *Journal of Clinical Endocrinology and Metabolism*, the study reported that vitamin D_3 is about 87 per cent more effective than vitamin D_2 at increasing circulating vitamin D levels.

Researchers from the University of Surrey in the United Kingdom analyzed data from seven randomized controlled trials that directly compared the efficacy of vitamin D_2 and vitamin D_3 on circulating vitamin D levels. This first-ever systematic review and meta-analysis, published in a 2012 issue of the *American Journal of Clinical Nutrition*, reported that vitamin D_3 is more successful at increasing circulating vitamin D levels than vitamin D_2.

Finally, scientists at the University of Otago in New Zealand conducted a randomized, double-blind, placebo-controlled trial to evaluate the potency of daily 1,000-IU doses of vitamin D_2 and vitamin D_3 in ninety-five healthy adults over twenty-five weeks beginning at the end of summer 2009. They concluded that daily supplementation of 1,000 IU of vitamin D_3 was more effective than vitamin D_2 in maintaining circulating vitamin D levels during the winter. Furthermore, the researchers discovered that a daily intake of 1,000 IU of vitamin D_2 decreased circulating vitamin D levels. Their findings were reported in a 2012 edition of the *British Journal of Nutrition*.

Summary

The majority of medical studies conclude that vitamin D_3 is more effective in defending your life than vitamin D_2. Knowing the availability of vegan vitamin D_3 supplements, I do not see any reason why someone would take vitamin D_2, a less potent supplement. If your healthcare practitioner prescribes vitamin D, beware that you will be getting vitamin D_2 (at least in the United States). When buying a vitamin D supplement, check the ingredients on the label to ensure you are selecting cholecalciferol—the real vitamin D_3! ☀

Chapter 5

Vitamin D₃'s Partners

Vitamin D_3 does not work alone in the body. Other vitamins and minerals partner (act as co-factors) with activated vitamin D_3 to perform the essential functions explained in Chapter 3. Fat-soluble vitamin K_2 is dependent upon vitamins A and D_3's functions. Minerals including calcium and magnesium also team up with vitamin D_3. Before I further address vitamin D_3's associates, I caution you to carefully read this chapter. The fact that specific vitamins and minerals function effectively with vitamin D_3 does not mean that you should begin (or increase) taking supplements of these nutrients without considering your medical profile or consulting your healthcare practitioner.

Vitamin A

Vitamins D_3 and A regulate genetic activity that causes cells to make proteins required by water-soluble vitamins and minerals. The functions of these vitamins comprise the foundation of our health. Vitamin A deficiency is rare as common animal and plant foods contain this nutrient. Therefore, supplementation is usually unnecessary. When cod liver oil or retinol supplements such as retinyl acetate and retinyl palmitate are consumed, vitamin A toxicity may occur. Excess vitamin A in the body may create havoc because it denies vitamin D_3 from influencing the genetic activity described above. Vitamin A supplementation may obviate the wonderful benefits of vitamin D_3. Please be careful!

Vitamin K_2

Vitamins D_3 and K_2 partner to build and maintain strong bones and teeth as well as fight cardiovascular disease (CVD). Vitamin D_3's functions include regulating calcium absorption in the intestines to maintain bones and dental health. However, once calcium enters the blood stream, vitamin D_3 relinquishes control of the mineral's destination to a little-known nutrient called vitamin K_2 that moves calcium out of the arteries and into the bones and teeth.

Let's take a look at vitamin K_2 and how it complements vitamin D_3. Like vitamins A and D_3, vitamin K_2 belongs to a family of fat-soluble nutrients. Two distinct forms of vitamin K offer medical value: phylloquinone and menaquinone.

Phylloquinone or vitamin K_1 is present in all green plants that acquire energy from sunlight. Green leafy vegetables including spinach, kale, collards, broccoli, and brussel sprouts abound with vitamin K_1. Clotting blood is primarily vitamin K_1's life-saving benefit. Since vitamin K_1 constantly recycles in the body, deficiency is rare.

Menaquinone or vitamin K_2 differs greatly from K_1. There are two forms of vitamin K_2: menaquinone-4 (MK-4) found in grass-fed animal protein including meat, egg yolk, butter, some cheeses, and calf's liver. A fermented soybean called natto, commonly consumed in Japan, is abundant in a more potent form of vitamin K_2 called menaquinone-7 (MK-7).

Health benefits of adequate vitamin K_2 levels include potential prevention of osteoporosis, arterial plaque, and dental cavities. Vitamin K_2 moves calcium to the bones and teeth, as well as sweeps calcium from soft tissue lining such as arteries. Specifically, vitamin K_2 activates proteins (osteocalcin and MGP [matrix gla protein]) produced by vitamin D_3 that facilitate moving calcium to where it belongs: the bones and teeth.

Low vitamin K_2 levels, however, are common. First, vitamin K_2 receptors need regular replenishment, as they are not recycled in the body. Second, the vitamin's natural sources are lacking in most diets. When insufficient vitamin K_2 is in the blood stream, calcium can linger along arterial pathways potentially causing calcification, the process whereby calcium deposits form plaque accumulating in the cardiovascular system.

Supplementing with adequate vitamin D_3 and K_2 balances calcium metabolism. The word "balance" is important: one can enjoy optimal vitamin D_3 levels but unknowingly have a vitamin K_2 deficiency, a potential recipe for CVD development. Unless you ingest grass-fed animal products or natto on a regular basis, consider taking a daily K_2 supplement. Some experts recommend a daily dose between 100 and 120 mcg. (I take a daily 90-mcg vitamin K_2 [MK-7] soft gel containing natto.) WARNING: Anticoagulant medications (blood thinners such as warfarin) block the action of vitamin K. If you are taking blood-thinning medication, please check with your healthcare professional before adding any form of vitamin K to your body.

Calcium

Calcium is the best known of vitamin D_3's partners. Vitamin D_3 regulates this essential mineral's absorption in the intestines so it can contribute to bone and tooth health. Calcium supplementation, however, is a topic of debate in the medical community. While calcium is essential to the bones and teeth, this mineral can linger throughout the body, potentially causing calcification in soft tissue including the kidneys and cardiovascular system. If you are taking a calcium supplement or a combined vitamin D_3 and calcium pill, you may want to reconsider. Personally, I no longer take calcium supplements because my serum calcium level is within normal range. Furthermore, I have opted to consume a daily vitamin K_2 supplement (see above paragraph) to increase the likelihood that the calcium in my body is moved to my bones and teeth.

Magnesium

Magnesium is essential to vitamin D_3's metabolism and absorption. Low magnesium levels may impair the conversion of circulating vitamin D_3 to the activated form, denying your body of vitamin D_3's amazing health benefits. An abundance of medical literature indicates that magnesium is one of the most important elements in maintaining health. Its benefits include energy production, protection of the nervous system, improvement of muscle function, and a decrease in cardiovascular disease risk.

In today's world of fast food and pharmaceutical drugs, magnesium deficiency is common. Many diets lack natural sources of magnesium including green leafy vegetables, legumes, seeds, and nuts. Furthermore, prolific use of prescription drugs such as antibiotics, proton pump inhibitors (some anti-acid medications), and osteoporosis medications contribute to depletion of the body's magnesium levels. A daily magnesium supplement of at least 200 mg may boost your levels of this important mineral.

Summary

Vitamin D_3 functions in concert with fat-soluble vitamins A and K_2 as well as a number of minerals. To reap the benefits of this amazing nutrient, you should be aware of vitamin D_3's vitamin and mineral partners. The next part of this book presents an in-depth look at how vitamin D_3 supplementation may prevent or treat a variety of medical conditions. ☀

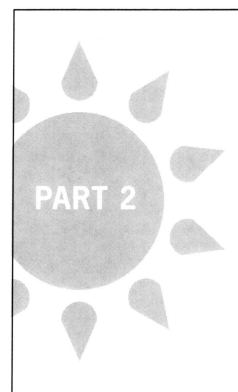

PART 2

Benefits of Vitamin D$_3$

Benefits of Vitamin D₃

Sitting in bumper-to-bumper Los Angeles traffic, I noticed Hollywood High School—known for its expansive list of celebrity graduates—nestled on the corner of Sunset Boulevard and Highland Avenue. Taking the opportunity to peek at the iconic school, I peered through a line of sun-drenched palm trees bordering the campus. Traffic suddenly burst forward, affording only a glimpse of the Science Building, specifically the concrete border above one of the windows. When my eyes caught the boldly-stated inscription, "Science Is Truth Found Out," I thought about many scientists who have researched vitamin D_3 and realized that its health benefits reach far beyond bone health.

"Science *Is* Truth Found Out"

The truth is all musculoskeletal beings require adequate amounts of vitamin D_3 to develop and maintain good health. Science has demonstrated that vitamin D_3 possesses mechanisms of action that may prevent and/or treat a wide variety of medical conditions including:

Asthma
Autism
Body aches and pain
Bone disease (including osteoporosis, and fractures)
Cancer (including breast, colon, and prostate)
Cardiovascular disease
Common cold
Dental issues
Diabetes (types 1 and 2)
Digestive conditions (including Crohn's disease, IBS, and colitis)
Eye conditions (including macular degeneration)
Female conditions (including PMS and uterine fibroids)
Genetic aging
Hearing loss
Inflammation
Influenza (including H1N1)
Lupus
Mental disorders (including Alzheimer's and dementia)
Migraines
Multiple sclerosis
Muscle weakening
Non-Hodgkin's lymphoma
Parkinson's disease
Pregnancy and newborn issues
Pulmonary disease (including COPD and cystic fibrosis)
Rheumatoid Arthritis
Skin conditions (including acne, dermatitis, eczema, and psoriasis)
Testosterone deficiency
Thyroid disorders

The scientific evidence about vitamin D₃'s benefits is enlightening and, in some cases, compelling. At the time of publication, a plethora of vitamin D studies were under way. I can only envision additional emerging information that will further strengthen the connection between vitamin D₃ and health.

Conflicting Studies. When analyzing scientific studies, it is important to carefully examine the data to avoid misleading conclusions. For example, the November 2008 issue of the *Journal of the National Cancer Institute* reported clinical trial results that concluded: a) vitamin D supplementation did not decrease invasive breast cancer risk, and b) circulating vitamin D₃ levels were not associated with breast cancer risk. This summary contradicts the positive conclusions of the majority of medical research linking vitamin D₃ and breast cancer, at least in part, because the trial only administered a low daily dose—400 IU—of vitamin D₃ to its participants. Such a woefully deficient dose would not be expected to lower the risk of breast or any other form of cancer.

Chapter 6

Athletic Performance

Since I was a child, I have been an avid sports fan. My early love of baseball eventually cascaded into a passion with an array of team sports. Can you imagine my excitement—while researching this book—to learn that there is yet another potential "good news story" about vitamin D_3: legally enhancing athletic performance!

First, let me make clear that I am not talking about using vitamin D_3 for illegal purposes to improve athletic prowess. We have heard the stories about professional athletes taking performance-enhancing "drugs" banned by their governing organizations. These reported cases frequently focus on the supplementation of steroids such as testosterone and human growth hormone, substances of which young men and women naturally possess sufficient levels. As you have learned from this book, the majority of people—at any age—suffer from inadequate levels of vitamin D_3 primarily because of sun avoidance.

Second, the purpose of vitamin D_3 supplementation for athletes is to attain adequate levels. You may recall that vitamin

D_3 supplements, or cholecalciferol, are nutrients. After being processed by our liver and kidneys, cholecaliferol converts to the active form of vitamin D_3, or calcitriol. Calcitriol is a steroid hormone that partners with millions of vitamin D receptors in our cells, tissues, and organs to affect a wide variety of beneficial actions in our bodies, including the repair and maintenance of muscle tissue. When a circulating vitamin D_3 test confirms that an individual is deficient in vitamin D_3 and, consequently, this person supplements to attain adequate levels, evidence suggests that vitamin D_3 consumption can improve athletic performance.

A Professional Hockey Team Supplements with Vitamin D_3 and Wins the Stanley Cup!

In May 2010, John J. Cannell, MD, founder and executive director of the Vitamin D Council, announced anecdotal evidence that the improved performance of the National Hockey League's Chicago Blackhawks team could be a possible consequence of vitamin D_3 supplementation. Chicago's professional hockey team had not competed in a playoff game since 2002. According to Dr. Cannell's sources, team physicians for the Chicago Blackhawks commenced diagnosing and treating all players for vitamin D_3 deficiency around 2008. The majority of the players reportedly took daily doses of 5,000 IU of vitamin D_3. Sources also asserted that the Chicago Blackhawks benefited from fewer colds and cases of influenza, as well as a decrease in "repetitive use" injuries. Subsequently, the Chicago Blackhawks played significantly better than the previous six seasons. In fact, they won professional hockey's top prize: the Stanley Cup!

Other Connections between Vitamin D$_3$ and Athletic Performance

Researchers from Liverpool John Moores University (LJMU) studied circulating vitamin D$_3$ levels of twenty professional soccer ("football" outside the United States) players on the legendary Liverpool FC team. The players' circulating vitamin D$_3$ levels in August 2010 were about 40 ng/mL, a value significantly higher than the national average of the United Kingdom (UK). This relatively high measurement most likely was a result of the players spending a busy World Cup season outdoors and closer to the equator than their club's home latitudinal location of 53 degrees North. When the players' circulating vitamin D$_3$ levels were measured four months later (in December), the researchers learned the levels plummeted about 50 percent to an average of 21 ng/mL! The study, published in the August 2012 edition of the *Journal Applied Physiology, Nutrition and Metabolism*, suggests the importance of adequate circulating vitamin D$_3$ levels to maintain muscle function.

A placebo-controlled trial conducted by LJMU researchers examined the effects of a daily 5,000 IU vitamin D$_3$ supplementation on musculoskeletal performance of sixty-one UK-based professional athletes during an eight-week period. The study, published in an October 2012 online issue of the *Journal of Sports Science and Medicine*, revealed a significant increase in the 10-meter sprint and vertical jump performances by the athletes who supplemented with vitamin D$_3$. The LJMU researchers concluded that inadequate circulating vitamin D$_3$ levels are "detrimental to musculoskeletal performance in athletes" and urged future studies of vitamin D_3's effects on larger athletic groups.

Researchers presented a study at the American Orthopaedic Society for Sports Medicine's July 2011 annual meeting that connects vitamin D_3 deficiency to an increased risk of muscle injuries in professional athletes. They measured circulating vitamin D_3 levels of eighty-nine members of one National Football League team in spring 2010 as part of routine pre-season evaluations. The team provided information about the players who lost playing time due to muscle injuries. The mean circulating value of the sixteen players who suffered muscle injuries was a woefully low 19.9 ng/mL.

The December 2009 issue of *Runner's World* included an article about the potential for higher vitamin D levels to boost athletic performance. Author Karen Asp surmised that U.S. marathon record holder, Deena Kastor, sustained a bone fracture in her foot during a 2008 Beijing Olympic competition, owing to a vitamin D deficiency discovered after the race. Kastor's blood reportedly contained sufficient levels of calcium but lacked the circulating vitamin D_3 levels to effectively absorb the bone-essential mineral. The *Runner's World* story acknowledged that the majority of runners—as is the majority of the population—are vitamin D deficient, and cited a number of recent studies that accentuate vitamin D_3's benefit to athletic performance.

Dr. Cannell and colleagues exhaustively pored through worldwide medical literature to ascertain vitamin D_3's relationship with athletic performance. They published their findings in the

May 2009 issue of *Medicine & Science in Sports and Fitness*, and concluded peak athletic performance might be achieved when individuals attain optimal vitamin D_3 levels at least 50 ng/mL.

According to a British study included in the February 2009 edition of the *Journal of Clinical Endocrinology and Metabolism*, adolescent females with higher circulating vitamin D_3 levels demonstrated the ability to jump quicker and faster than pubertal females in the same age (twelve- to fourteen-year-old) group. The researchers concluded that vitamin D_3 "was significantly associated with muscle power and force in adolescent girls."

A review in the December 2008 issue of *Molecular Aspects of Medicine* titled, "Emerging Roles of Vitamin D: More Reasons to Address Widespread Vitamin D Insufficiency," indicated that vitamin D enhances muscular strength. Conversely, low vitamin D_3 levels might increase the risk of bone fractures and other sports-related injuries.

Summary

Echoing other vitamin D_3 advocates, I truly hope that vitamin D_3 supplementation regimens will be implemented in amateur and professional sports programs to help players minimize injuries and improve performance. Vitamin D_3 and athleticism equate to better balance, speed, reaction time, and muscle strength. Go team! ☀

Chapter 7

Autism

When a pregnant woman is asked if she is hoping for a boy or girl, her inevitable response is similar to, "I only care that my baby is healthy." Many expectant mothers do their best to have healthy babies by leading wholesome lifestyles and following doctors' orders. Nonetheless, millions of babies are born with birth defects including autism, a developmental disorder possibly caused by genetic damage.

The symptoms and severity of autism vary widely. Autistic symptoms usually appear during the child's first three years. Autistic children have difficulties with social interaction and communication, as well as exhibit repetitive behavior or obsessive interests. Some autistic children's symptoms improve with treatment and age. However, children whose communication skills regress, usually before the age of three, may be at risk of developing epilepsy or seizure-like brain activity. Furthermore, some autistic adolescents may become depressed or demonstrate behavioral problems.

Autism often is a life-long disability that affects the quality of life of autistic persons and their families. Real-world issues include special education, social support, self-sufficiency, and employability. Money also is a big concern. Medical treatment primarily comprises years of taking expensive prescription drugs. The economic cost of raising an autistic child in 2006 was staggering: up to $3.2 million over the individual's lifetime! In comparison, the typical cost to raise a healthy child for seventeen years was about $222,000 in 2006. These daunting figures only have increased since 2006.

Who is at Risk to Develop Autism?

Autism is on the rise. Over the past two decades, an alarming number of children—in the United States and other industrialized countries—have been diagnosed with autism. According to a U.S. government study published in a 2011 issue of the journal *Pediatrics*, the prevalence of developmental disabilities—led by autism—in U.S. children increased 17 percent in the past decade! Approximately one in 110 children born in the United States is diagnosed with autism. Males are five times more likely to develop autism than females.

Why are autistic cases increasing? Is there a correlation between vitamin D_3 and autism? A growing number of scientists agree that vitamin D_3 deficiency plays an important role in autism development. Esteemed vitamin D expert John J. Cannell, MD, espouses a theory that a significant relationship exists between vitamin D_3 and the rising incidence of autism. Dr. Cannell believes that as people have become "sun-phobic" over the past decades, the prevalence of autism has risen. In addition, prenatal vitamins—the "gold standard" of nutritional supplements for pregnant women—only contain a small dose of vitamin D_3, usually between 400 and 800 IU, an inadequate amount to protect against brain defects in developing fetuses.

Dr. Cannell acknowledges his theory is "readily susceptible to rigorous testing." He believes his theory that vitamin D_3 reduces the risk of autism is strong enough that "[the possibility] deserves immediate attempts to disprove it."

Two doctors in the Middle East investigated the relationship between circulating vitamin D_3 and autism severity by studying fifty autistic children between five- and twelve-years-old and comparing them with thirty healthy youngsters. The researchers found that the autistic subjects had significantly lower vitamin D_3 levels than the healthy kids (14 ng/mL vs. 33 ng/mL). They also discovered *inter alia* that the circulating vitamin D_3 levels of the autistic children were directly correlated with autism severity. The findings of the study were published in the August 17, 2012 issue of the *Journal of Neuroinflammation*.

Let's look at the connection between autism and vitamin D_3. Autism is a developmental brain disorder, probably caused—at least in part—by genetic damage. Every cell in the brain has vitamin D_3 receptors (VDRs). The receptors control genes that influence brain development. In order to control genes in the brain, the VDRs must be turned on by receiving adequate activated vitamin D_3. Without vitamin D_3 to activate its receptors, the brain does not properly develop. According to Cannell, the brain levels of activated vitamin D_3 "directly depend on the amount of vitamin D the mother makes in her skin or puts in her mouth."

How Can Vitamin D$_3$ Prevent Autism?

Autism may possibly be prevented by women having adequate circulating vitamin D$_3$ levels before and during their pregnancies, as well as during lactation. In addition to vitamin D$_3$'s role in gene expression, this essential nutrient possesses antiviral, antibacterial, and anti-inflammatory properties that protect against infections, free radicals, etc., that could be incurred during pregnancy.

Dr. Cannell's theory holds credence with many scientists. While we await results of the "rigorous testing" invited by Dr. Cannell, why allow this brain disorder to develop in fetuses, newborns, and infants? For little—if any—risk, women who could be or could become pregnant should seriously consider getting tested for their circulating vitamin D$_3$ level and ensure, in concert with their practitioners, that their vitamin D$_3$ supplementation is adequate. According to Dr. Cannell's Vitamin D Council website, pregnant and nursing women require 6,000 IU per day of vitamin D$_3$ supplements during pregnancy for optimal births and during lactation in order to provide infants sufficient vitamin D$_3$. If you hope to conceive soon, or have recently become pregnant, it is not too late to get your vitamin D$_3$ levels up to par.

The subject of vitamin D$_3$'s influence on autism remains one of Dr. Cannell's top priorities. In June 2011, I participated in a vitamin D workshop led by Dr. Cannell. The association between vitamin D_3 and autism was one of the forum's main subjects. Dr. Cannell discussed how a simple solution such as an adequate vitamin D_3 supplement may prevent autism in most newborn children. Dr. Cannell suggested pregnant and lactating women take a daily vitamin D_3 dose of 6,000 IU to protect their children from developing autism. Ideally, he emphasized the importance of both biological partners to build and maintain their vitamin D_3 levels.

How Can Vitamin D_3 Treat Autism?

Anecdotal evidence suggests a possible association between vitamin D_3 and treatment of autistic persons. At the time of this writing, however, I am unaware of medical studies that examine this relationship. Nonetheless, as the executive director of the Vitamin D Council, Dr. Cannell receives many letters from parents of autistic children. The progress described by these parents is heartwarming, yet subjective, evidence that sufficient vitamin D_3 supplementation can diminish autism symptoms in both children and young adults.

For example, a mother of a four-year-old autistic boy reported to Dr. Cannell that after only two months of daily vitamin D_3 5,000 IU supplementation, her young child exhibited significant behavioral improvements including more eye contact, smiling, listening, and social interacting.

Dr. Cannell received a letter from a mother of a nineteen-year-old son with regressive autism, who had suffered years from a dizzying array of debilitating ailments. The young man, whose initial circulating vitamin D_3 was a paltry 17mg/mL, demonstrated temper tantrums, other behavioral outbursts, and mood swings as well as severely lacked verbal communication skills. After he took a daily dose of 6,000 IU of vitamin D_3 for several weeks, the young adult could not "stop talking." His mother joyfully reported that her son was not only using complex grammar but he began singing!

Subsequently, the mother increased her son's daily dose to 10,000 IU with the intent of raising his circulating vitamin D_3 level. Dr. Cannell surmised that "10,000 IU/day will not harm autistic adults and it may help..." He suggested the mother obtain another blood test in two months for her son and adjust his daily dose to attain a circulating vitamin D_3 level in the 80-100 ng/mL range. By the way, the changes in the nineteen-year-old's behavior were so amazing that his mother videotaped "before" and "after" segments as proof of his incredible improvement.

Autistic parents' stories provide encouraging information about the potential of vitamin D_3's effectiveness in treating autism. Dr. Cannell believes that vitamin D_3 supplementation regulates the appropriate genes in the brain of autistic persons to improve brain function. Too few data exist, however, to know if activated vitamin D_3 can permanently improve autistic symptoms.

In 2011, Dr. Cannell opened a free public clinic to treat vitamin D_3 deficiency in autistic children. Sponsored by the Vitamin D Council, the clinic includes a consultation, an autism assessment scale, blood tests, and if needed, vitamin D_3 supplements.

Vitamin D$_3$ Supplementation's Potential Value in Preventing and Treating Autism

The link between autism and vitamin D$_3$ appears to be genuine. The lower a biological couple's circulating vitamin D$_3$ levels, the more likely their child will develop autism. The encouraging news is that adequate vitamin D$_3$ supplementation by biological parents prior to conception may prevent autism in their children. Furthermore, a possibility also exists that vitamin D$_3$ supplements may treat autistic individuals.

Why wait for the results of years-long "rigorous testing" by the medical community? Time is of the essence to prevent the development of autism in fetuses, infants, and children. Couples who are planning to conceive a baby should seriously consider getting tested for their circulating vitamin D$_3$ level and ensure, in concert with their practitioners, that their vitamin D$_3$ supplementation is adequate. ☀

Chapter 8

Cancer

For centuries, society has regarded cancer as a condition both respected and feared. Many people expect that we are genetically and environmentally disposed to contracting some form of cancer during our lifetimes. Our fears are not unfounded. The United Nations' cancer research agency estimated that cancer will kill over 13.2 million people a year by 2030, almost twice the number who died from the disease in 2008. Furthermore, the American Cancer Society has labeled cancer as the world's top "economic killer." In 2008, cancer's global price tag was approximately $895 billion.

We should not acquiesce to cancer's escalating death rate and economic costs. Vitamin D_3 has the potential to prevent and treat different types of cancers. Let's look at how vitamin D_3 works to prevent the development and growth of malignant cells.

The adult human body comprises about 100 trillion cells. Many of these cells include vitamin D receptors that receive, store, and in some cases, produce activated vitamin

D_3. Activated vitamin D_3 influences cells to grow—and die— normally. When cells do not behave normally, they can proliferate and become "rogue" cells that offer an inviting home for cancer development. If the body has sufficient activated vitamin D_3 stored in its cells, vitamin D_3 will incite natural cell death. Vitamin D_3's capability to affect natural cell death negates the opportunity for cancer cells to proliferate, develop into a tumor, and spread to other parts of the body. This fact alone should encourage everyone to ensure their vitamin D_3 levels are adequate!

Scientific evidence has linked the importance of vitamin D_3 to cancer prevention. A landmark study published in a 2007 edition of the *American Journal of Clinical Nutrition* revealed a protective effect for vitamin D_3 and calcium against cancer in women. Dr. Joan M. Lappe and her Creighton University colleagues conducted a four-year, randomized controlled trial (RCT) to determine the effectiveness of calcium and vitamin D_3, as well as calcium alone, on the incidences of all types of cancer in postmenopausal women. This highly acclaimed RCT was the first of its type to demonstrate that increasing circulating vitamin D_3 can positively affect the overall risk for cancer.

Activated vitamin D_3's process of natural cell death holds great promise in the prevention and treatment of many types of cancer. The link between vitamin D_3 and three prevalent types of cancer—breast, colorectal, and prostate—is addressed in this chapter.

BREAST CANCER

Many women truly fear breast cancer. They worry about getting breast cancer themselves, as well as the possibility of their grandmothers, mothers, sisters, children, aunts, cousins, and friends being diagnosed with it. Some women who are diagnosed with malignancy in one breast opt for the excision of both breasts to eliminate a possible occurrence of the dreaded disease. Furthermore, some females who are genetically predisposed to breast cancer undergo a double mastectomy to obviate the threat of developing breast cancer.

American women's trepidation is well-justified. The United States has the highest rate of breast cancer in the world. The American Cancer Society estimated that in 2012 about 226,870 women would be diagnosed with new cases of invasive breast cancer, and approximately 39,510 females will die from the disease.[1] In addition, about 63,300 women will be diagnosed with the earliest stage of breast cancer called carcinoma in situ, a non-invasive form.

For decades, chemotherapy has been conventional medicine's primary response to treating breast cancer. Chemotherapy, however, does not discriminate between healthy and cancerous cells, and accelerates bone loss. After one of my dear aunts underwent years of grueling chemotherapy treatments for breast cancer, she succumbed to the devastating disease in 2008. As the specter of breast cancer lingers over many women, I thought, "There has to be a much better answer to breast cancer prevention

---

[1] Men also can develop breast cancer. In 2009, 440 males in the United States reportedly died of breast cancer.

and treatment." Now I believe there is—at least a partial—safe, inexpensive, and effective response to breast cancer: attainment and maintenance of sufficient circulating vitamin D_3 levels. I am strongly encouraged by medical evidence that maintaining sufficient vitamin D_3 levels could not only reduce the risk of developing breast cancer but could treat at least early-stage breast cancer patients.

How Vitamin D_3 Can Prevent Breast Cancer

Breast (mammary gland) cells contain a high level of vitamin D receptors (VDRs) that receive and produce activated vitamin D_3. If these VDRs are sufficiently active, they exude anti-cancer effects by: demonstrating anti-inflammatory effects; regulating cellular differentiation, proliferation, and natural death in breast tissue; and suppressing tumor growth. If the VDRs in the breast tissue are not working at their optimal level, breast cancer may develop.

Columbia University researchers conducted a population-based, case-controlled study, published in a 2009 issue of the journal *Cancer Prevention Research*, which examined the association between breast cancer and circulating vitamin D_3. They found an inverse relationship with circulating vitamin D_3 levels and the risk of breast cancer. The study data suggest that the optimal circulating vitamin D_3 level for breast cancer prevention should be 40 ng/mL or greater. The researchers concluded that the study results add to a growing body of evidence that adequate, activated vitamin D_3 (stored in the VDRs) "may prevent breast cancer development."

University of California San Diego (UCSD) scientists examined eleven observational studies about the association between breast cancer incidence and circulating vitamin D_3. Their findings, published in a 2011 issue of *Anticancer Research*, concluded people with circulating vitamin D_3 levels of 47ng/mL or more enjoyed a 50 percent lower risk of developing breast cancer.

In 2011, researchers from the Stanford University School of Medicine published a paper in the *Annual Review of Pharmacology and Toxicology* that examined vitamin D_3 as an anti-cancer agent. Vitamin D_3's mechanisms of action: cell regulation; anti-inflammatory effects; tumor growth suppression; and reduction in estrogen production may prevent or treat breast cancer.

A team of vitamin D researchers evaluated a wide range of "scientific evidence" that provided "compelling evidence" of vitamin D's protective role in the risk of developing breast cancer. Their findings, published in a 2012 issue of the journal *Dermato-Endocrinology*, concluded that vitamin D_3 plays an "important role in the prevention of breast cancer." The scientists characterized vitamin D_3 supplementation as a "low cost, effective, and safe intervention strategy for breast cancer prevention that should be implemented without delay."

For decades, epidemiological research has indicated a correlation between sunlight exposure and incidences of breast cancer.

University of South Carolina researchers studied the number of breast cancer cases in relation to the distance from the equator of population residence. They studied almost three million breast cancer cases diagnosed in sixty-four global regions over periods ranging from two to fifty-three years. The investigators determined that the farther women live from the equator, the more likely they will develop breast cancer. Results of the study, published in a 2010 issue of *Breast Cancer Research and Treatment*, conclude that breast cancer development occurs predictably with the seasons. In other words, breast cancer incidences peak near spring and fall equinoxes, and decline near summer and winter solstices.

In 1990, Cedric Garland and his brother Frank, renowned researchers at the UCSD's School of Medicine, and colleagues, demonstrated the foresight to suggest not only that an individual's vitamin D level from exposure to sunlight rays could be associated with breast cancer risk, but the differences in ultraviolet light striking the U.S. population could account for the significant regional differences in breast cancer mortality!

Ed Gorham, PhD, in concert with the Garland brothers at UCSD's School of Medicine, conducted a 1990 study of Soviet women that revealed lower rates of breast cancer in regions where there was more sunlight exposure. Dr. Gorham also indicated findings that nations within 20 degrees of the equator have less breast cancer cases than countries farther from the equator.

How Vitamin D$_3$ Can Treat Breast Cancer

Vitamin D$_3$ receptors in breast tissue cells receive and produce activated vitamin D$_3$. This fact alone suggests that vitamin D$_3$ has the potential to treat at least the early stages of breast cancer. Medical research also indicates vitamin D$_3$ may play a role in treating breast cancer.

Norwegian researchers studied the association between circulating vitamin D$_3$ levels and risk of death in cancer survivors including 251 breast cancer patients. The breast cancer survivors with the highest circulating vitamin D$_3$ levels enjoyed the lowest risk of death. Their findings, published in a 2012 issue of the journal *Cancer Causes and Control*, concluded that higher levels of circulating vitamin D$_3$ increased the rate of survival for breast cancer patients.

Researchers at the Mayo Clinic in Jacksonville, Florida conducted a medical literature review that was published in a 2010 issue of the journal *Nutrition*. Although data suggests an association between adequate vitamin D$_3$ levels and improved cancer prognosis, the researchers surmised that adequate vitamin D$_3$ levels may benefit breast cancer survivors by improving bone mineral density, mood, and quality of life. The Mayo Clinic scientists recommended breast cancer survivors maintain adequate vitamin D$_3$ levels "throughout their lifetime."

University of Sao Paulo researchers examined breast cancer tissue of fifty Brazilian women to understand how vitamin D$_3$ inhibits the growth of breast cancer cells. The investigators learned that activated vitamin D$_3$ receptors impede the formulation of blood vessel growth around malignant breast tumors. Published in a 2002 issue of the *Brazilian Journal of Medical and Biological Research*, the study demonstrated the anti-proliferative functions of vitamin D$_3$.

In the July 2008 issue of the *American Journal of Clinical Nutrition*, experts from the Fred Hutchison Cancer Research Center in Seattle, Washington who sought to better understand circulating vitamin D_3 levels in breast cancer survivors published their findings. Of the 790 multiethnic, breast cancer survivors from western Washington State, Los Angeles County, and New Mexico evaluated in the study, the vitamin D_3 levels of about 75 per cent of the women were deficient. In other words, the research indicated a correlation between breast cancer and vitamin D_3 levels. The scientists concluded that the prevalence of vitamin D_3 deficiency was high in breast cancer survivors, and suggested clinicians consider monitoring—and appropriately treating—vitamin D_3 levels in breast cancer patients.

Summary

Medical research strongly suggests that adequate vitamin D_3 levels may prevent the development of breast cancer. In addition, recent studies indicate that vitamin D_3 supplementation may help treat breast cancer survivors. Since attaining and maintaining adequate vitamin D_3 levels, my confidence about a significantly diminished risk of developing breast cancer has soared.

COLORECTAL CANCER

Colorectal cancer (commonly referred to as "colon cancer") is a silent killer that begins in the colon or the rectum. According to the American Cancer Society, colorectal cancer is the second-leading cause of cancer-related deaths in the United States. Almost 50,000 persons were predicted to die from this disease during 2011.

In the majority of people, colorectal cancer develops slowly over several years with symptoms that can be interpreted as common complaints. Prior to the development of colorectal cancer, tissue growth usually starts as a non-cancerous polyp on the inner lining of the colon or rectum. Although many polyps are benign, they can become cancerous as result of inflammation. Once the cancer develops in a polyp, cancer cells can eventually grow into the wall of the colon or rectum. Entry of cancer cells into the colon or rectum wall can facilitate the spread of cancer into blood or lymph vessels. Hence, cancer originating in the colon or rectum can spread to different areas of the body.

Thanks to improved screening techniques and treatment protocols, the death rate from colorectal cancer is steadily declining. Nonetheless, adequate vitamin D_3 status may play a significant role to stop colorectal cancer before it develops. Evidence also suggests vitamin D_3 can treat at least the early stages of colorectal cancer.

How Vitamin D_3 Can Prevent Colorectal cancer

Over 95 percent of colorectal cancers—called adenocarcinomas—begin in the colorectal mucosal cells that form mucus-producing glands to lubricate the lining of the colon and rectum. The mucosal cells also contain vitamin D_3 receptors that receive and produce activated vitamin D_3.

Most medical experts agree that chronic inflammation can cause normal cells to go awry—hence, become cancerous. Not surprisingly, inflammatory bowel diseases including Crohn's disease and ulcerative colitis cause chronic inflammation of the colon. Once again, vitamin D_3's anti-inflammatory mechanisms help prevent inflammation—one of the initial conditions that could lead to the development of colorectal cancer.

Over thirty years ago vitamin D pioneers and brothers Cedric and Frank Garland proposed "vitamin D as a protective factor against colon cancer" to the medical community. Their 1980 hypothesis, published in the *International Journal of Epidemiology*, arose from examining the geographical distribution of colon cancer deaths in the United States. The Garland brothers theorized that colorectal cancer mortality rates were highest in areas where people were exposed to the least amount of natural sunlight.

Turning the clock ahead twenty-five years, the Garland brothers and other esteemed vitamin D researchers investigated the appropriate vitamin D_3 intake that could significantly decrease the risk of developing colorectal cancer. They concluded that a daily dose of 1,000 IU vitamin D_3 was associated with a 50 percent lower risk of developing colorectal cancer. The researchers encouraged "public health action" to increase the daily intake of vitamin D_3 to protect against the potentially deadly form of cancer. Since the publication of this research in a 2005 issue of the *Journal of Steroid Biochemistry and Molecular Biology*, subsequent studies further support the strong relationship between vitamin D_3 and the lower risk associated with the development of colorectal cancer.

How Vitamin D₃ Can Treat Colorectal cancer

We know that vitamin D receptors in the colon and rectum's mucosal cells both receive and produce activated vitamin D_3. This fact alone suggests that vitamin D_3 has the potential to treat at least the early stages of colorectal cancer.

Recent scientific findings garner optimism for vitamin D_3's potential role in treating initial stages of colorectal cancer:

Norwegian researchers studied the association between circulating vitamin D_3 levels and risk of death in cancer survivors including fifty-two colorectal cancer patients. The colorectal cancer survivors with the highest circulating vitamin D_3 levels enjoyed the lowest risk of death. Their findings, published in a 2012 issue of the journal *Cancer Causes and Control*, concluded that higher levels of circulating vitamin D_3 increased the rate of survival for colorectal cancer patients.

In August 2011, researchers at the Vall d'Hebron Institute of Oncology in Barcelona, Spain announced that vitamin D_3 supplementation may be an effective treatment in the early stages of colon cancer. Studying mice and human colon cells, the researchers concluded that VDRs in colon cells—primarily unaffected by tumor growth—slow the action of a key carcinogenic protein called beta-catenin.

According to vitamin D expert Michael F. Holick, PhD, MD, cancer patients with adequate circulating vitamin D_3 status respond better to chemotherapy. In addition, these patients have reduced tumor growth and less spreading of the disease to other parts of the body.

Summary

Adequate vitamin D_3 status may significantly reduce the risk of developing colorectal cancer. Vitamin D_3 status also may have the potential to treat colorectal cancer during its initial stages. Obviously, additional scientific research needs to be done. Nonetheless, why risk getting this horrible cancer, when, for pennies a day, you can add vitamin D_3 to your body to help prevent the disease.

PROSTATE CANCER

Prostate cancer is yet another silent but lethal cancer. Cancer of the prostate—a reproductive gland found only in men—is the second-leading cause of cancer deaths of males in the United States. According to the American Cancer Society (ACS), over 33,000 men were expected to die of prostate cancer in 2011.

More than 240,000 cases of prostate cancer arise each year in the United States. Unlike the decrease in the number of colorectal cancer cases, the incidence of prostate cancer has increased in the United States.

In the majority of men, the cancer develops slowly when the genes in the prostate cells change abnormally. The exact cause of prostate cancer remains unknown.

Age is a predominant risk factor for developing prostate cancer. About two of every three cases are diagnosed in men over the age of sixty-five. Prostate cancer is more common in African-American men than in males of other ethnicities. Another noteworthy ACS statistic encompasses the geographic location of prostate cancer victims: the disease is most common in North America and northwestern Europe.

Do these statistics ring a familiar bell? Let's see: people with darker skin color and living in northern latitudes pose a risk of vitamin D_3 deficiency. Adequate vitamin D_3 status may play a significant role to stop prostate cancer before it begins. Evidence also suggests vitamin D_3 may treat at least early stages of prostate cancer.

How Vitamin D_3 Can Prevent Prostate Cancer

Prostate gland cells contain vitamin D receptors (VDRs) that receive and produce activated vitamin D_3. If VDRs are sufficiently active, they exude a number of anti-cancer effects including fighting inflammation and regulating gene expression to promote natural cell death. A sampling of medical studies supporting the connection between vitamin D_3 and prostate cancer are:

In 1990, University of North Carolina researchers hypothesized in the journal *Anticancer Research* that vitamin D deficiency may be a significant risk for the development of prostate cancer. Fortunately, their hypothesis triggered a plethora of medical studies supporting vitamin D_3's positive role in preventing prostate cancer.

In 2003, eminent vitamin D expert Michael Holick and a Boston University School of Medicine colleague published a study examining the association between vitamin D_3 and prostate cancer. The researchers concluded that decreased sun exposure or vitamin D_3 deficiency was directly related to an increased risk of prostate cancer. They suggested "adequate vitamin D nutrition should be a priority for men of all ages."

Researchers in Spain studied ninety-one prostate cancer patients to evaluate, inter alia, circulating vitamin D_3 levels. Their findings, published in a 2011 issue of the journal *Sociedad Espanola de Endocrinologia y Nutricion*, concluded vitamin D_3 deficiency was "highly prevalent" among the cancer patients.

A 2011 study examined prostate cancer incidence rates in seventy local government areas of Australia to determine the relationship between prostate cancer cases with average "solar radiation" exposure in non-urban regions of the country. The researchers concluded that less UVB sun rays are associated with a high prostate cancer incidence in Australia.

How Vitamin D_3 Can Treat Prostate Cancer

Vitamin D receptors (VDRs) in the prostate cells both receive and produce activated vitamin D_3. This fact alone suggests that vitamin D_3 has the potential to treat at least the early stages of prostate cancer. Medical research suggests vitamin D_3 may play a role in treating prostate cancer.

Vitamin D expert Michael F. Holick, PhD, MD, and a Boston University colleague concluded in a 2003 study that cancer cells in the prostate respond to VDRs by increasing their death and decreasing their growth and invasiveness. The researchers' findings support the use of vitamin D therapy as a treatment for prostate cancer.

Professor Reinhold Vieth, PhD, of the University of Toronto presented evidence at a 2004 conference at the National Institutes of Health that vitamin D_3 can help treat some cancers, including prostate cancer. He and his colleagues administered a daily dose of 2,000 IU vitamin D_3 to fifteen men with advanced prostate cancer. Despite the relatively low vitamin D_3 dose, the majority of the patients demonstrated an improved PSA (prostate-specific antigen) value, a measurement of the spread of prostate cancer.

Harvard University researchers examined malignant tissue of 841 prostate cancer patients to understand the role of VDR function in prostate tumors in relation to the risk of lethal prostate cancer. Their findings, published in a 2011 edition of the *Journal of Clinical Oncology*, indicated that prostate cancer patients with lower vitamin D_3 levels are more likely to succumb to the disease than patients who have higher vitamin D_3 status.

Summary

Adequate vitamin D_3 status may significantly reduce the risk of developing prostate cancer. Vitamin D_3 status also may have the potential to treat prostate cancer during its initial stages. The ACS projects that more than 33,000 men in the United States will die annually from prostate cancer. Sufficient vitamin D_3 supplementation may save many of these lives. Why risk getting this cancer? For pennies a day, you can add vitamin D_3 to your body to help prevent this potential deadly disease. ☀

Chapter 9

Cardiovascular Disease

Cardiovascular disease (CVD) causes the greatest number of deaths of Americans. According to a 2010 American Heart Association (AHA) statistical report, "every minute, someone in the United States dies from a heart-related event." Heart disease[2] is the No. 1 killer of American females.

CVD comprises any medical condition affecting the heart and arteries. Examples of CVD include: high blood pressure (hypertension); peripheral arterial disease; blocked arteries (coronary heart disease); stroke; heart attack (myocardial infarction); chest pain (angina); hardening of the arteries (atherosclerosis); blood clotting (thrombosis); inflammatory heart diseases; and, vein inflammation (phlebitis). High blood pressure, the most common CVD in the United States, is often a prelude to more serious CVD such as coronary heart disease, atherosclerosis, stroke, and heart attack.

---

[2] The expression "heart disease" refers to a number of CVD including coronary heart (or artery) disease, myocardial infarction, and heart failure.

Diagnosis of some CVD types is more difficult in women than men. Females are more likely to develop a CVD at a less detectable level—in tiny microvessels—than men, who tend to get blockages in the larger blood vessels of the heart, according to Kathy Magliato, MD, a Los Angeles cardiothoracic surgeon. About 50 percent of women do not experience chest pain, the most apparent CVD symptom. Other CVD warning signs include: shortness of breath; persistent, unexplainable fatigue; indigestion; nausea; arm pain (especially in the left arm); and jaw or throat pain.

In 2010, heart disease cost the United States approximately $316.4 billion! This staggering figure includes the cost of health care services, medications, and lost productivity.

Who is at Risk to Develop CVD?

The majority of American adults are at risk of developing at least one type of CVD. Lifestyle choices contribute to a higher risk of developing CVD as well as specific medical conditions. Nine of ten heart disease patients have at least one risk factor. According to the AHA, these risk factors include: high blood pressure (a CVD that can cause other CVDs); high cholesterol; diabetes; chronic kidney disease; unhealthy diet; smoking; alcohol use; overweightness and obesity; and physical inactivity.

The risk of developing CVD is not all about disease and lifestyle. Another CVD risk factor is inadequate vitamin D_3. Over three decades ago, Professor Robert Scragg of the University of Auckland reported in the *International Journal of Epidemiology* that the incidence of CVD tends to be seasonal. On the one hand, CVD cases are more common during the winter when fewer UVB rays correlate with lower vitamin D_3. On the other hand, during the summer months CVD occurs less frequently when more UVB light boosts higher vitamin D_3.

Researchers at the Intermountain Medical Center in Murray, Utah examined 41,504 patient records with at least one circulating vitamin D_3 level for the prevalence of vitamin D_3 deficiency and CVD. Low vitamin D_3 readings were "highly associated" with a number of CVDs including coronary heart disease, heart attacks, strokes, and death. The scientists' observations, reported in the *American Journal of Cardiology* in 2010, indicated a likely association between vitamin D_3 and CVDs.

Published in 2009, a Swedish study of 40,000 women over eleven years concluded that females who enjoyed "more active sun exposure" were at 30 percent lower risk of developing blood clotting in the veins and arteries than women who had little contact with sunlight.

How Can Vitamin D_3 Prevent CVD?

Vitamin D_3's powerful functions may decrease the risk of developing CVD. The cardiovascular system hosts vitamin D_3 in a big way. The heart muscle cells and the blood vessels' smooth muscle cells contain the key enzyme that converts circulating vitamin D_3 to activated vitamin D_3. In addition, vitamin D receptors (VDR) reside in the heart muscle cells, the smooth muscle cells in the blood vessel walls, and the lining of the blood vessels. The omnipresence of VDR in the cardiovascular system results in activated vitamin D_3 that promotes heart and vascular health by minimizing plaque development, reducing inflammation, and enhancing muscle strength.

Vitamin D_3 partners with vitamin K_2 to clean the arteries and blood vessels by moving calcium to your bones and teeth rather than to cardiovascular tissues. Adequate vitamin D_3 may prevent CVDs exacerbated by calcium deposits that form plaque: hardening of the arteries (atherosclerosis); peripheral artery disease; coronary heart disease; and blood clotting (thrombosis).

Vitamin D_3's anti-inflammatory properties fight viruses and bacteria. Adequate vitamin D_3 levels may reduce inflammatory heart diseases such as myocarditis, pericarditis, and endocarditis. Phlebitis, or vein inflammation, is another type of CVD that may be prevented by circulating vitamin D_3.

Activated vitamin D_3 maintains and strengthens the heart muscle and artery muscle cells. The heart comprises mostly muscle so a weak heart can lead to a host of serious conditions including heart failure.

A blocked artery or a ruptured blood vessel in the brain can cause a stroke. Once again, vitamin D_3's capability to sweep calcium out of arteries, fight inflammation in blood vessels, and maintain muscle strength in blood vessel walls may reduce the risk of a stroke.

How Can Vitamin D_3 Treat CVD?

At of the time of this writing, I am unaware of any studies to examine vitamin D_3's role in treatment of CVDs. Given what the scientific community knows about vitamin D_3's activities within the cardiovascular system, I think it is likely that adequate circulating vitamin D_3 levels may treat CVD, at least in some cases.

Vitamin D_3 Supplementation's Potential Value in Fighting CVD

Sufficient vitamin D_3 supplementation may combat CVDs. Vitamin D_3's functions, including moving calcium to the bones and teeth; fighting bacteria and viruses; and strengthening heart and arterial muscles, play an important role in cardiovascular health.

Observational studies indicate that persons with higher circulating vitamin D_3 enjoy a lower risk of developing or dying from CVDs. At the time of this writing, I am unaware of any randomized controlled trials (RCTs) that either demonstrate or disprove that greater initial vitamin D_3 lowers the incidences of CVDs. I also am not cognizant of RCTs concerning vitamin D_3 treatment of individuals with CVD.

What is the probability of funding RCTs to study the effect of vitamin D_3—a non-patented nutrient—on cardiovascular health? Apparently quite low. Would you prefer to wait years for the results of possible RCTs? Or would you prefer easily attaining (and maintaining) adequate vitamin D_3 levels that could decrease your odds of developing or dying from the No. 1 killer of American adults? ☀

Chapter 10

The Common Cold

The dreaded common cold usually strikes at the worst time: vacation; school events; visiting family and friends; an important meeting; air travel; formal presentation or speech, etc. The cold indeed is "common," as the U.S. population suffers from about 500 million colds a year! In the United States most adults can expect to catch a cold two to four times annually. Children are more susceptible, contracting colds about six to ten times a year. The common cold drains at least $40 billion from the U.S. economy each year! About half of the cost is attributed to lost time from work. The remaining costs are derived from medical care, over-the-counter treatments, and prescription medicine.

What is the Common Cold?

The common cold is an upper respiratory viral infection. Although over 200 viruses can cause colds, rhinovirus is the most common virus that inflicts the highly contagious illness. Symptoms of the common cold include runny nose, sneezing, nasal obstruction, sinus congestion, sore throat, and coughing. A cold can last up to two weeks. Some colds turn into bronchitis, a lung infection of which about 90 percent are caused by a virus.

On both sides of the globe, the common cold occurs more frequently during the autumn and winter seasons, when exposure to UVB sunlight is the lowest. For years, the conventional thinking was that people caught colds more often in colder seasons because people's activities occur more frequently indoors. For example, children returning to confining classrooms in the fall season are more apt to develop colds. Recent thinking however attributes the higher risk of colds to less sunlight exposure and vitamin D_3 intake. Vitamin D_3's antiviral and anti-inflammatory properties may lower the risk of contracting the common cold.

How Can Vitamin D_3 Prevent the Common Cold?

Vitamin D_3 may lower the likelihood of contracting the common cold and other upper respiratory tract infections (URTIs) by producing proteins (cathelicidin and defensins) that reduce the risk of viral infections. In addition, vitamin D_3's anti-inflammatory properties fight viral infections.

Results of a randomized controlled trial published in a 2012 issue of the journal *Pediatrics* support vitamin D_3's capability to prevent URTIs. A team of researchers, led by Carlos A. Camargo, Jr., MD, from Massachusetts General Hospital in Boston, studied 247 third- and fourth-grade Mongolian students to understand how vitamin D_3 supplementation may affect the incidences of acute respiratory infections. Mongolia's capital,

Ulaanbaatar, was selected because of its highly cold climate and latitude similar to northern states in the United States.

At the beginning of the study, circulating vitamin D_3 levels of the children averaged a woefully low 7 ng/mL. More than half (143) of the children received daily milk fortified with 300 IU of vitamin D_3. After three months, the control group's circulating vitamin D_3 levels were unchanged. However, the children who supplemented daily with 300 IU of vitamin D_3 averaged circulating levels of 19 ng/mL – almost triple their circulating values only three months prior to participation in the trial. Moreover, the children who received vitamin D_3-fortified milk enjoyed 50 per cent fewer colds than the control group!

Dr. Jim Bartley, a head and neck surgeon in Auckland, New Zealand, reviewed literature about the influence of vitamin D on immunity and URTIs. His study, published in a 2010 issue of the *Journal of Laryngology and Otolaryngology*, concluded that "vitamin D appears to play an important role of the innate immunity in the upper respiratory tract."

An encouraging study of 18,883 American adults and adolescents, led by Adit Ginde, MD, MPH, and published in 2009, examined the association between vitamin D_3 levels in the blood and URTIs. Characterizing the relationship between vitamin D_3 and URTIs as "robust," the study's authors concluded that people with lowest blood vitamin D_3 levels had significantly more cases of the common cold or influenza than those individuals with the highest vitamin D_3 levels.

How Can Vitamin D$_3$ Treat the Common Cold?

As of this writing, I am unaware of any reported studies of treating the common cold with vitamin D$_3$. Some medical professionals have suggested taking high doses of vitamin D$_3$ at the beginning of a cold to reduce the severity and duration of the common cold. However, each person reacts differently to vitamin D$_3$ supplementation. Significantly increasing one's dosing could still take two to three weeks for circulating vitamin D$_3$ levels to increase. In any event, high vitamin D$_3$ doses could potentially decrease the risk of the common cold turning into bronchitis, or worse, pneumonia.

Vitamin D$_3$ Supplementation's Potential Value in Combating the Common Cold

Given the medical community's recent understanding of vitamin D$_3$'s anti-inflammatory and antiviral properties, adequate vitamin D$_3$ supplementation may prevent the common cold. Ongoing scientific research will likely uncover additional evidence of vitamin D$_3$'s value of protecting against cold viruses.

Hopefully, optimal vitamin D$_3$ levels will improve health-related quality of life by helping us avoid getting the costly common cold. Prior to achieving an adequate vitamin D$_3$ level, I typically developed three to four colds a year. Since enjoying a consistently optimal vitamin D$_3$ level, I have only suffered one annual cold. Furthermore, during a seven-week period I flew a number of times across many time zones, and did not contract a cold or any illness—a welcome "first" for me! ☀

Chapter 11

Dental Health

Let's add improved dental health to the list of benefits reaped by vitamin D$_3$ supplementation! Do you know that an astonishing 25 percent of Americans over the age of sixty-five have no teeth, according to the Centers for Disease Control and Prevention? In addition, the National Institute of Dental and Craniofacial Research reported that about 58 percent of Americans fifty and older have fewer than twenty-one teeth (the normal number of teeth is thirty-two)!

Medical research indicates that your vitamin D$_3$ level correlates to the health of your teeth and gums. Keeping your teeth and gums strong also benefits the health of other parts of your body. In turn, your dental health directly relates to the wellness of key organs, most notably your heart, as well as your overall oral health. In addition to regular preventive visits to your dentist, supplementing with vitamin D$_3$ potentially could decrease your number of dental ailments including loose teeth, cavities, and periodontal, or gum, disease. Fewer dental issues mean fewer visits to the dentist chair and more financial savings!

You may be thinking, *teeth and gums? How does achieving and maintaining vitamin D₃ sufficiency benefit the condition of my teeth and gums?* If you recall, active vitamin D_3 has significant bone-strengthening and anti-inflammatory properties. Although teeth are not bones, your jawbone, or the alveolar bone, supports your gums and teeth. Hence, excellent oral bone health is important not only to preserve your teeth but also to keep them healthy!

Vitamin D Supports Tooth Retention and Strength

A 2001 study conducted by Boston University's Goldman School of Dental Medicine examined tooth loss in 145 healthy adults aged sixty-five years or older over a three-year, randomized, placebo-controlled trial to ascertain the effect of vitamin D and calcium supplementation on bone loss in the hip. The researchers' subjects also underwent a two-year follow-up study after discontinuing their trial supplements. The Boston University researchers concluded that vitamin D and calcium supplementation have a "beneficial effect on tooth retention."

In his 2010 book, *Power of Vitamin D*, Sarfraz Zaidi, MD, shares a couple of anecdotal stories about vitamin D's positive effect on dental health. First, after his patients' vitamin D_3 levels were "optimal," they reported to Dr. Zaidi that their dentists complimented them on the excellent condition of their teeth. Second, Zaidi endured sharp pain in one of his molar teeth. His dentist diagnosed the tooth as cracked, yet had no answer to the cause of the fracture. However, after Zaidi began taking daily doses of 8,000 IUs of vitamin D_3, his dentist marveled at the increased strength of Dr. Zaidi's teeth—no more dental fractures for him!

Vitamin D Decreases Tooth Decay

The protective effect of vitamin D_3 on tooth cavities has been known—at least indirectly—since the 1930s. According to his 2010 book, *The Vitamin D Solution*, renowned vitamin D expert, Michael F. Holick, PhD, MD, discusses a connection between sunlight exposure and the occurrence of tooth decay when a decades-old, ecological study concluded that "more sunlight exposure correlated with fewer cavities."

On account of its protective anti-inflammatory properties, vitamin D_3 supplementation assists your body's immune system to defend against bad bacteria and inflammation throughout your body. Therefore, maintaining an optimal circulating vitamin D_3 level induces the production of a protein, called cathelicidin, which counters bacterial infections in your mouth.

Vitamin D May Reduce Susceptibility to Gum Disease

Gum, or periodontal, disease is a common inflammatory condition that can cause tooth loss. Similar to its role in preventing tooth decay or loss, vitamin D_3's anti-inflammatory properties promote the manufacturing of the cathelicidin protein to fight bacterial infections in your mouth.

A Boston University Goldman School of Dental Medicine study, led by Thomas Dietrich, MD, D. MD, MPh, and published in a 2005 issue of the *American Journal of Clinical Nutrition*, evaluated the relationship between circulating vitamin D_3 levels and gingivitis, the most common form of gum disease. The researchers analyzed data from over 77,000 teeth in 6,700 never-smokers between ages thirteen- and ninety-years-old. The study concluded that vitamin D_3's anti-inflammatory effects may reduce susceptibility to gingivitis.

In 2009, Japanese scientists from the Nihon University School of Medicine in Tokyo studied the function of activated vitamin D receptors. They concluded that vitamin D_3 has the potential to be useful in the prevention and treatment of periodontal disease.

Researchers at the Saint Louis University Center for Advanced Dental Education in Missouri examined fifty-one dental patients in periodontal maintenance programs who took up to 1,000 IU daily doses of vitamin D_3 and calcium (about 1,700 mg) supplements. They concluded that these patients enjoyed better periodontal health compared to subjects not supplementing with these nutrients. One year later, the researchers conducted a follow-up study on the same patients that indicated a "modest positive effect on periodontal health." The study's findings—published in the first 2011 issue of the *Journal of Periodontology*—suggest that vitamin D_3 may positively affect periodontal heath, and called for randomized clinical trials to better ascertain the effects of vitamin D_3 on gum disease.

Vitamin D$_3$ Supplementation: The Sooner, the Better

It's probably never too late to begin vitamin D$_3$ supplementation in response to dental problems (or most health issues). However, the earlier in your life that you supplement with vitamin D$_3$, the better for your body as well as for the oral health of any children you plan to bring into the world. Why? According to a recent study conducted at the University of North Carolina, approximately 40 percent of pregnant women suffer from periodontal disease. Unfortunately, these mothers will pass this oral condition—in addition to other health issues—to their newborns. Conversely, pregnant women who are "vitamin D$_3$ sufficient" most often will contribute those benefits derived from vitamin D$_3$—including a healthy mouth—to their children. In addition, most prenatal vitamins contain only a small dose of vitamin D$_3$ (usually 400 IU). Vitamin D experts recommend that pregnant women, as well as infants, toddlers, and adolescents, supplement with vitamin D$_3$. ☀

Chapter 12

Diabetes

Diabetes mellitus—a group of diseases involving high blood sugar—affects more than 220 million persons worldwide, according to the World Health Organization (WHO). About 3.4 million persons die annually from the disease. The WHO predicts deaths from diabetes mellitus to double by 2030.

Over 10 percent of diabetics live in the United States. In 2010, the Centers for Disease Control and Prevention (CDC) estimated that about 24 million Americans have developed the disease. The CDC also predicted that new cases of diabetes will increase at least threefold by the middle of the twenty-first century.[3] The American Diabetes Association estimates the total cost associated with diabetes mellitus in the United States is more than $174 billion per year.

There are two major forms of diabetes mellitus: insulin-dependent Type 1 and lifestyle-induced Type 2. Each disease type and its association with vitamin D_3 are discussed below.

---

[3] The calculation includes an estimate of persons who are diabetic but are undiagnosed.

Type 1 Diabetes

Type 1 diabetes is a chronic autoimmune disease where the pancreas is unable to make insulin in its beta islet cells. The body's immune system attacks and destroys the pancreatic beta islet cells until insulin can no longer be produced. Insulin, a vital hormone, regulates blood sugar (glucose) levels in muscle and other tissue cells to help control energy. The lack of insulin creates elevated blood sugar.

Affecting about 5 percent of diabetics, type 1 diabetes usually occurs during childhood or adolescence but can strike at any age. Once type 1 diabetes has developed, it never goes away. Type 1's onset translates to a forever regimen: measuring blood sugar at least four times a day, injecting or pumping insulin as needed, monitoring carbohydrate intake, and exercising.

Many scientific studies have examined vitamin D_3's potential association with type 1 diabetes. A 2011 study funded by the Juvenile Diabetes Research Foundation supported the possibility that vitamin D_3 supplementation could play a role in preventing type 1 diabetes. Renowned vitamin D researcher Dr. Cedric Garland of the University of California San Diego discovered that type 1 diabetes is rare near the equator where its inhabitants enjoy year-round abundant UVB sunlight. He also found the prevalence of the disease increases the farther people live from the equator.

How Can Vitamin D_3 Prevent Type 1 Diabetes?

Vitamin D_3 has the potential to prevent type 1 diabetes. The pancreatic beta islet cells, that make insulin, contain vitamin

D receptors (VDR) that receive and produce activated vitamin D_3! So what does this mean? Activated vitamin D_3 protects the beta islet cells by reducing the production of cytokines, substances that destroy beta islet cells, and may prevent the development of type 1 diabetes.

One of the most significant studies about the association of vitamin D_3 and prevention of type 1 diabetes was published in a 2001 issue of the prestigious British journal *Lancet*. Researchers studied over 10,000 Finnish children who had received a "regular" 2,000 IU dose of vitamin D_3 since their birth in 1966. Over thirty years later scientists determined who in the birth-cohort study had been diagnosed with type 1 diabetes. They learned that vitamin D_3 supplementation reduced the risk of type 1 diabetes by about 80 percent!

Nestled in the Arctic region, Finland endures lengthy "vitamin D winters." Nonetheless, in 1975, the recommended daily allowance (RDA) of vitamin D_3 for infants in Finland was decreased from 2,000 IU to 1,000 IU. In 1992, Finnish officials further reduced infants' RDA for vitamin D_3 to a paltry 400 IU! This drastic reduction of recommended vitamin D_3 reportedly was based on the observation that sufficient vitamin D_3 is contained in a teaspoon of cod liver oil to prevent rickets. Is it any surprise that the rate of type 1 diabetes development in Finland has soared over the past decades?

According to the Vitamin D Council website, Dr. Cannell indicates that "the risk of type 1 diabetes may be reduced" by adhering to specific guidelines: a) pregnant women should have a circulating vitamin D_3 level above 30-40ng/mL;

b) infants should obtain 1,000-2,000 IU of vitamin D_3 by breast milk or supplementation; and c) parents should ensure their infants maintain a circulating vitamin D_3 level above 30 ng/mL. Dr. Cannell notes "further research is needed to confirm these values."

How Can Vitamin D_3 Treat Type 1 Diabetes?

At the time of this writing, I am unaware of vitamin D_3's capability to treat type 1 diabetes. The "Cardiovascular Disease" chapter mentions type 1 diabetes as a risk factor for developing cardiovascular disease (CVD). Therefore, people with type 1 diabetes may wish to maintain sufficient circulating vitamin D_3 levels to reduce their CVD risk.

Vitamin D_3 Supplementation's Potential Value in Fighting Type 1 Diabetes

Adequate vitamin D_3 levels in pregnant women, lactating mothers, and infants may indeed significantly reduce the risk of type 1 diabetes. If you plan to have children, you can wait about ten years for the results of further studies, or hop on the vitamin D_3 express before it's too late!

Type 2 Diabetes

Type 2 diabetes is a lifestyle-induced disease where increased body weight causes problems in the pancreas and intestines. As you gain too much weight, your body begins to resist insulin, causing the pancreas to make high levels of insulin to maintain normal blood sugar levels. The overworked pancreas begins to fail to the point where it cannot make enough insulin to maintain normal blood sugar levels. Further exacerbating the process, the intestines decrease their production of hormones, called incretins, which regulate insulin release and control satiety (a feeling of fullness). People who have low levels of incretins tend to eat more and gain more weight. This "domino effect" results in a condition called "insulin resistance." Insulin resistance can lead to the development of type 2 diabetes.

Affecting about 95 percent of diabetics, type 2 diabetes usually occurs during adulthood but is becoming common in teenagers. Obesity is a primary risk factor for developing type 2 diabetes. Unlike type 1 diabetes, your lifestyle (or changes to) can prevent and treat type 2 diabetes.

How Can Vitamin D₃ Prevent Type 2 Diabetes?

A healthy lifestyle is the best approach to preventing type 2 diabetes. An important aspect of a healthy lifestyle is maintaining your weight in the normal range for your gender, age, height, musculoskeletal frame, and genetic disposition. Obesity is strongly linked to the onset of type 2 diabetes.

So, how can vitamin D_3 prevent type 2 diabetes? Vitamin D_3 is fat-soluble, meaning it is absorbed by, and stored in, fat cells. The more body fat you have, the less vitamin D_3 is available for pancreatic beta islet and other cells to regulate insulin production. Hence, lower vitamin D_3 status—as a potential result of obesity—can increase the likelihood of developing type 2 diabetes. By increasing your vitamin D_3 status, you may decrease the likelihood of getting type 2 diabetes. Make sense?

Recent studies about the link between vitamin D_3 and type 2 diabetes suggest that vitamin D_3 status may affect the onset of type 2 diabetes.

Researchers at the University of Melbourne studied 5,200 Australian adult men and women over a five-year period to ascertain if circulating vitamin D_3 levels could predict the development of type 2 diabetes. The study, published in a 2011 issue of *Diabetes Care*, concluded that higher circulating vitamin D_3 levels were associated with a "significantly reduced risk" of type 2 diabetes.

In 2010 and 2011, Tufts Medical Center published studies about the relationship between circulating vitamin D_3 and type 2 diabetes. For example, the researchers conducted a sixteen-week, randomized controlled trial of pre-diabetic adults, half of whom supplemented with vitamin D_3. The pancreatic beta islet cells' function of the vitamin D_3 subjects improved 300 times by taking a daily 2,000 IU dose over four months!

How Can Vitamin D_3 Treat Type 2 Diabetes?

Vitamin D_3 directly influences the pancreatic cells where insulin is made. Attaining and maintaining an adequate vitamin D_3 status may help treat type 2 diabetes by regulating insulin production. The food industry is recognizing this theory as well. For example, fortification of commercial yogurt with vitamin D_3 to combat, in part, type 2 diabetes has become common.

Vitamin D₃ Supplementation's Potential Value in Fighting Type 2 Diabetes

Sufficient vitamin D_3 levels may prevent the lifestyle-induced, type 2 diabetes in persons who are overweight and have abnormal, fasting blood glucose readings. If you think you are on the path toward type 2 diabetes, consider adding vitamin D_3 supplementation as part of changing to a healthier lifestyle.

Summary

Vitamin D_3 plays a significant role in both types of diabetes mellitus. We know that vitamin D_3 deficiency is related to impaired pancreatic beta islet cells and insulin resistance. Adequate vitamin D_3 status may contribute to the prevention of type 1 diabetes. Sufficient vitamin D_3 status may help to prevent and treat type 2 diabetes.

Why acquiesce to projected diabetes figures tripling by 2050? Let's strive to reduce the number of diabetes cases by a third or more by the mid-twenty-first century! ☀

Chapter 13

Genetic Aging

Would you like to live a longer, healthier life? Medical research indicates that vitamin D_3 may play a key role in the genetic aging process.

Before we look at how vitamin D_3 may affect genetic aging, let's review some basics: The nucleus of every cell in our body includes forty-six pairs of genetic strands called chromosomes. Chromosomes contain DNA (deoxyribonucleic acid), hereditary molecules encoded with genetic instructions essential to the body's development and function. The end of each chromosome contains a telomere (visualize a cap on each end of a shoelace). Telomeres protect vital DNA in the chromosomes. When chromosomes normally divide, or differentiate in response to oxidative stress, the telomeres gradually fray until the cells become dysfunctional or expire, potentially causing adverse health conditions and aging.

The biological age of our cells can be measured by the length of our telomeres that become shorter as we age chronologically and biologically. A human embryo has the longest telomeres. A newborn baby has telomeres shorter than upon conception. A child's telomeres are shorter than an infant's. And so forth. As adults, we can be certain that the length of our telomeres decreases as we grow older.

Telomere length also can predict the risk of developing aging-related diseases. Inflammation is a major culprit for turning our biological clocks ahead of their time because it may shorten telomeres. When telomeres are exposed to inflammation, they become shorter. The shorter the telomere, the faster aging occurs. Conversely, the longer the telomere, the slower aging takes place. Lengthier telomeres are associated with longer, healthier life!

How can we benefit from having telomeres that are longer than our chronological age? By attaining and maintaining adequate circulating vitamin D_3 levels that will provide activated vitamin D_3 to the vitamin D receptors (VDRs) attached to our DNA. In other words, activated vitamin D_3 influences our genetic code.

A landmark study, published in the October 2010 edition of the journal *Genome Research*, accentuates the significance of vitamin D_3's powerful gene regulation. University of Oxford researchers discovered 2,776 binding sites for VDRs along the length of a human genome (a complete set of chromosomes). Moreover, they found that these VDR-binding sites were unusually concentrated near a number of genes associated with predisposition to autoimmune diseases including multiple sclerosis, lupus, Crohn's disease, type 1 diabetes, and rheumatoid arthritis, as well as some types of cancer, including colorectal! The research also revealed that vitamin D_3 significantly affected the activity of 229 genes including those associated with susceptibility to some of the autoimmune diseases cited above.

Another vitamin D_3 mechanism of action encompasses regulation of cellular functions, including cell division, cell differentiation, cell proliferation, and apoptosis. An additional benefit of vitamin D_3 is its anti-inflammatory mechanism of action. As a powerful inhibitor of inflammation, vitamin D_3 reduces stress on our cells, potentially slowing telomere shortening.

Compelling evidence, published in a 2007 issue of the *American Journal of Clinical Nutrition*, suggests that vitamin D_3 may reduce the rate of telomere shortening. Researchers from King's College London School of Medicine compared the telomere lengths of 2,160 female twins, ages eighteen to seventy-nine, with their circulating vitamin D_3 levels. The higher their vitamin D_3 levels, the longer their telomeres. The difference between the highest and lowest circulating vitamin D_3 levels equated to five years of telomere, or biological, aging. In other words, a sixty-year-old woman with higher circulating vitamin D_3 levels may enjoy a biological age of fifty-five years!

Can Vitamin D_3 Slow Genetic Aging?

The connection between vitamin D_3 and genetic aging is real. Vitamin D_3's mechanisms of action, including gene expression, cell regulation, and anti-inflammatory functions may influence biological aging as well as the likelihood of developing autoimmune disease and possibly some types of cancer. Additional scientific research will further uncover how vitamin D_3's genetic role can help defend your life. ☀

Chapter 14

Influenza

In Chapter 1 of this book, I noted the general angst as information about the spread of the new—and potentially fatal—H1N1 virus, or swine flu, circled the globe. The anxiety associated with catching the disease was well-founded as many people did not possess a pre-existing immunity. About eighteen months after the announcement of the beginning of the H1N1 outbreak, the World Health Organization (WHO) announced the H1N1 pandemic ended and estimated that over 186,000 persons had died globally from the deadly virus. Nonetheless, WHO virus experts continue to encourage health authorities to remain vigilant for pandemics of other influenza strains. Furthermore, the WHO chief of global influenza program Sylvia Brand warned that viruses "are evolving" and "changing all the time." Medical history supports the WHO's admonition about the evolution and unpredictability of viruses. The H1N1 strain provides a recent example.

In addition to specialized influenza virus strains, every year many countries grapple with how to prevent, or at least minimize, seasonal influenza. So what should be done to prevent the human contraction of influenza viruses? For decades, the primary answer has been vaccines. Immunization treatment against influenza has been somewhat controversial owing to inter alia, the mercury content in the vaccine, and the guess work involved predicting the most likely strains to appear during the "flu season," thus adding uncertainty to the effectiveness of the vaccine.

It's that time of year again; signs advertising flu shots dot the commercial landscape. Retail pharmacy stores conveniently sell flu inoculations while shopping. Flu-shot kiosks at airports are common. Pharmaceutical companies produce flu vaccines in nasal-spray form for younger people and high-dose flu shots for older folks. When I think about this ambitious marketing campaign, my reaction is the same: adequate vitamin D_3 levels may protect us from influenza as effectively as flu vaccines.

The "flu" is a highly contagious, respiratory disease caused by a type (or strain) of influenza virus. Influenza A, the most common flu virus, usually prevails during the autumn and winter seasons when the least exposure to ultraviolet B sunlight occurs. Seasonal flu vaccines comprise a mixture of the most predictive influenza viruses. However, the effectiveness of flu immunization can be called into question because of the uncertainty about which flu strain will emerge during the season.

Activated vitamin D_3 has a profound impact on the immune system. Vitamin D_3's antiviral and anti-inflammatory functions may lower the risk of contracting or dying from influenza. To strengthen the immune system, activated vitamin D_3 produces two peptides called cathelicidin and defensin that combat viruses.

In addition, vitamin D_3 reduces the risk of mortality from the flu by decreasing the production of a pro-inflammatory protein called cytokine. The anti-inflammatory action of vitamin D_3 also inhibits the development of bacterial pneumonia that can develop from influenza and result in death.

John J. Cannell, MD, founder and executive director of the Vitamin D Council, advocates the connection between activated vitamin D_3 and influenza. In 2006, he and colleagues published a paper in the British journal *Epidemiology and Infections* that proposed low vitamin D_3 levels are why the flu occurs more often during the winter. They also suggested that adequate daily vitamin D_3 supplementation may reduce influenza symptoms. Subsequently, Dr. Cannell led a team of researchers who further examined vitamin D_3's mechanisms of action on epidemic influenza. Published in the February 2008 issue of the *Virology* journal, the researchers confirmed the association between vitamin D_3 deficiency and the seasonality of influenza.

From December 2008 through March 2009, researchers conducted a randomized, double-blind, placebo-controlled trial involving over 300 Japanese schoolchildren. Children who took a daily 1,200 IU supplement of vitamin D_3 benefited from up to a 60 percent reduction in the influenza A infection rate during the darkest months of the year. Four times as many children in the placebo group developed the flu compared to the vitamin D_3 group. (Note: A daily dose of 1,200 IU is quite low compared to current recommendations of vitamin D experts.)

More than 186,000 persons died from the H1N1 "swine flu" (a strain of Influenza A) pandemic in 2009-10. Months after the initial outbreak of the virus, University of Virginia researchers published an article in the *Journal of Environmental Pathology, Toxicology and Oncology* strongly recommending that "all healthcare workers and patients be tested and treated for vitamin D deficiency to prevent" the spread of the H1N1 virus.

A 2012 article published in the journal *Critical Reviews in Microbiology* reviewed data from randomized, controlled clinical trials to examine the impact of vitamin D_3 supplementation in infectious diseases including influenza. The Dutch scientists indicated that vitamin D_3 supplementation may prevent or possibly treat influenza viruses, but noted that the optimal daily dosage regimen of vitamin D_3 has yet to be determined.

A study published in the September 27, 2012 issue of the *European Journal of Nutrition* examined laboratory results of the treatment of bronchial cells infected with influenza A virus, specifically the H1N1 strain, with vitamin D_3. The Indian researchers found that vitamin D_3 reduced the severity of H1N1 influenza.

Sales of vitamin D_3 supplements have dramatically increased over the past several years. For the first time in a decade, worldwide sales of influenza vaccines reportedly decreased over $4 billion in 2011. It is possible that vitamin D_3 awareness and consumption may have contributed to the decline in the flu vaccine markets. Given the medical community's understanding of vitamin D_3's antiviral and anti-inflammatory impact on the immune system, adequate vitamin D_3 intake may prevent influenza as well as potentially alleviate flu symptoms.

Last and perhaps not least, if you recall my story about sitting on a long flight next to a passenger who exhibited swine flu or influenza-like symptoms, I was not uncomfortable as I normally would be in this situation. Understanding that vitamin D_3 plays a key role by enhancing the immune system to protecting us against a wide array of diseases, I knew that my vitamin D_3 level was at least 50 ng/mL at the time. Having sufficient vitamin D_3 status improved the quality of my flight and I did not worry. I believed vitamin D_3 protected against H1N1 virus as well as other contagious diseases that most likely permeated through the airplane. ☀

Chapter 15

Multiple Sclerosis

Multiple sclerosis. The first time I heard of this incurable disease was when my mother told me that my dear cousin Judith Ann had developed the illness. I felt bad as I admired Judith Ann. She babysat me; was one of the first persons in our family to graduate from college; became a teacher; and married a U.S. Navy officer, Hugh Doyle. As a young girl modestly living in suburban Philadelphia, I viewed Judith Ann's life like a dream as her husband's career took her to exciting places such as New Zealand and San Diego.

As young adult, I was shocked to learn that Judith Ann, a mother of three children, had been diagnosed with multiple sclerosis. Despite enduring progressive damage to her nervous system, she courageously raised her family while Hugh was at sea. Judith Ann eventually was confined to a wheelchair. The debilitating nature of the disease caused Hugh, a Vietnam War veteran, to retire early to care for her. At the relatively young age of fifty-eight, Judith Ann died of complications caused by multiple sclerosis.

When I began researching vitamin D$_3$, I was encouraged to learn about its potential role in preventing and treating the disease that ended my cousin's life. This chapter was written in fond memory of Judith "Judy" Ann Armstrong Doyle.

What is Multiple Sclerosis?

Multiple sclerosis (MS) is an autoimmune disorder that damages the multiple layers of tissues, or the myelin sheath, that protect the nerves in the brain and spinal cord. On the one hand, when the sheath of tissues is intact, electrical impulses are carried through the nerves with accuracy and speed. On the other hand, when the myelin sheath becomes damaged, nerves do not conduct electrical impulses in a normal manner, resulting in a wide array of symptoms, ranging from numbness to partial blindness to brain damage. Primary progressive MS—the most lethal subtype of the disease—can be fatal.

Who is at Risk to Develop MS?

Approximately 400,000 people in the United States have been diagnosed with MS. Globally, more than 2.5 million persons are suffering from the disease. MS is at least two to three times more common in women, and usually begins between the ages of twenty and fifty.[4] The disease has been diagnosed more frequently in Caucasians of northern European descent than African Americans, Hispanics, or Asians.

---

[4]MS also can develop in children, teenagers, and older adults.

In 1868, a French neurologist reportedly identified MS for the first time. Almost a century and a half later, there still is no cure for this terrible disease! For decades, however, the medical community has suspected that where persons spend the first fifteen years of their lives affects their chances of developing MS. For example, people raised near the equator almost never develop MS. Do inadequate levels of vitamin D_3 cause MS? There is evidence to suggest that pregnant women with low circulating vitamin D_3 levels are at a greater risk to develop MS. Some researchers have surmised that vitamin D_3—the sunshine vitamin—could play a role in preventing and treating MS.

According to a study published in January 2011, University of Oxford researchers examined MS patterns in Scotland by studying hospital admissions throughout the country between 1997 and 2009. Subsequently, the researchers discovered a "highly significant relationship between MS-patient-linked admissions and latitude" across Scotland.

A Norwegian study, conducted by Trygre Holmoy of the University of Oslo's Medical Center, concluded that the risk of contracting MS "is associated with low vitamin D status prior to the disease." The study was electronically published on June 14, 2007, and appeared in a 2008 issue of *Medical Hypotheses*.

Medical studies of human subjects support the theory that women who develop MS have a vitamin D_3 deficiency. A study, led by Jeri Nieves, PhD of the Helen Hayes Hospital in West Haverstraw, New York, of eighty females with MS indicated that vitamin D_3 deficiency was prevalent in the majority of the subjects. The research was published in the September 1994 issue of *Neurology*.

How Can Vitamin D₃ Prevent MS?

To date, no cure for MS has been developed. The encouraging news is that vitamin D_3 may help to prevent the debilitating disease. Since the majority of people do not live in the equatorial region, perhaps the best MS prevention is for women of child-bearing age to enjoy optimal vitamin D_3 levels before becoming pregnant. While pregnant, mothers should ensure continued adequate vitamin D_3 intake. After childbirth, mothers—in concert with their healthcare providers—should ensure that their infants, toddlers, adolescents, and teenagers receive adequate vitamin D_3 supplementation.

Let's look at some compelling evidence that persons who have sufficient circulating vitamin D_3 levels enjoy a significant decreased risk of developing MS compared to individuals who have low vitamin D_3 levels:

From 1980 to 2001, the Harvard School of Public Health conducted two long-term studies of women to ascertain the protective effect of vitamin D_3 intake on the risk of developing MS. During the first study, known as the Nurses' Health Study, Harvard scientists followed 92,253 women from 1980 to 2000. The Nurses' Study II assessed 95,310 adult females from 1991 to 2001. The results of the two studies were published in a 1994 issue of *Neurology*. The studies, led by Kassandra L. Munger, concluded that vitamin D_3 intake has a positive effect on the risk of MS development in women. In addition, the studies demonstrated a 40 percent risk reduction of developing MS in nurses who took at least a daily dose of 400 IU of vitamin D_3 supplements. Despite the fact that a daily dose of 400 IUs is relatively small, the study demonstrated that even low-dose vitamin D_3 supplements have a protective effect against MS.

According to a study published in a December 2006 issue of the *Journal of the American Medical Association*, Harvard School of Public Health scientists partnered with associates at the Brigham and Women's Hospital and Harvard Medical School to examine whether circulating vitamin D_3 levels are associated with an MS risk. At the time of the study, the U.S. Department of Defense Serum Repository stored over seven million blood serum samples of U.S. military personnel. MS cases were identified through U.S. Army and Navy "physical disability databases for 1992 through 2004." A medical records review confirmed the MS diagnosis of the military personnel. Dr. Kassandra Munger, the leader of this study, and her team suggested that "high" levels of circulating vitamin D_3 "are associated with a lower risk of MS."

The January 2009 issue of *Multiple Sclerosis* includes a study, led by Dr. Jolijn Kragt of the VU Medical Center in Amsterdam, The Netherlands, which examined the role of vitamin D_3 in MS patients by analyzing vitamin D_3 levels of 103 MS patients and 110 healthy control individuals. The resultant data suggested that higher circulating vitamin D_3 levels "are associated with a lower incidence of MS and MS-related disability in women."

Previous medical studies have indicated that MS patients are born more often during the spring than in any other season. For years, the medical community has suspected that a seasonal risk factor exists for MS. According to a paper published in a February 2009 issue of *Public Library of Science (PloS) Genetics*, researchers from the University of Oxford and University of British Columbia suggested that a gene variant called HLA-DRB*1501 is associated with an increased risk of developing MS. And guess what? Vitamin D_3 influences how effectively the HLA-DRB*1501 gene variant works in the body. As we know, the amount of vitamin D_3 synthesized by UVB sunlight exposure fluctuates from season to season. Therefore, women who give birth during the spring carry the HLA-DRB*1501 gene variant and have low vitamin D_3 levels are probably more likely to produce children with a higher risk of developing MS.

The study's lead author, Dr. Sreeram Ramagopalan, has stated that adequate vitamin D_3 supplementation during pregnancies may decrease the risk of children developing MS in later life. The combination of carrying the HLA-DRB*1501 gene variant and lacking sufficient circulating vitamin D_3 levels possibly might impair the ability of the thymus, an immune system organ, to delete rogue T-cells, a type of white blood cells, that play an important role in maximizing the immune cells. The rogue cells would attack the body, causing a loss of vital tissue layers, or the myelin sheath, protecting the nerves in the brain and spinal cord. Hence, the autoimmune disease MS would develop. The scientists, however, acknowledged that future studies will be essential to better understand vitamin D_3's role in MS.

A February 2011 issue of the journal *Neurology* reported a ground-breaking study led by Robyn M. Lucas, PhD, and a team of her colleagues from the Australian National University in Canberra. For the first time a study was conducted to ascertain the effect of vitamin D_3 status and sun exposure on people who had recently experienced their first MS symptom, or initial demyelinating event (IDE), and had not been diagnosed with MS. IDE symptoms include visual disturbances, limb numbness, and dizziness. The Australian National University researchers compared 216 women and men aged eighteen to fifty-nine who had experienced an IDE to 395 individuals who exhibited no MS symptoms. The scientists matched the subjects' gender, age, and latitudes of residence. Dr. Lucas and her colleagues concluded that "high" circulating vitamin D_3 levels and sun exposure have a protective effect against the risk of developing MS. The researchers recommended that both vitamin D_3 levels and sun exposure "will need to be evaluated in clinical trials for multiple sclerosis prevention."

In October 2012, Australian and New Zealand scientists launched a ground-breaking, international clinical trial to determine if vitamin D_3 supplementation can prevent MS in people who have experienced their initial episode of MS-like symptoms, called Clinical Isolated Syndrome. During the four-year study the researchers also intend to ascertain the appropriate vitamin D_3 dosage to thwart the debilitating disease.

Queen Mary University of London researchers conducted a systematic review of data about 151,978 MS patients to ascertain the link between month and location of birth, and the risk of developing MS. They found that babies born in April had the highest risk of development of MS, and children born in October enjoyed the lowest risk of MS. The researchers also noted a direct correlation between the latitudinal location of expecting mothers and MS risk. The study, published electronically on November 14, 2012 by the *Journal of Neurology, Neurosurgery, and Psychiatry*, highly suggests the importance of maternal vitamin D_3 supplementation, at least during the winter season, and in countries where sunlight exposure is lowest between October and March.

Burgeoning research indicates a strong correlation between sufficient vitamin D_3 levels and MS prevention. The first step in prevention ideally would begin with child-bearing-age women. Subsequent actions would involve vitamin D_3 supplementation to attain optimal levels in infants, toddlers, adolescents, teenagers, and adults. In other words, everyone can increase their protection against debilitating diseases such as MS by taking a safe and inexpensive vitamin D_3 supplement on a daily basis.

How Can Vitamin D_3 Treat MS?

Vitamin D_3 and sunlight exposure may help to alleviate some MS symptoms. When an MS victim has high circulating vitamin D_3 levels, the patient's symptoms lessen. Conversely, MS symptoms intensify when the patient's circulating vitamin D_3 level is low. Sunlight exposure also affects how MS patients feel. During the winter season MS symptoms worsen. Furthermore, medical examinations of brain lesions indicate an increase of these lesions during winter. Studies published in the twenty-first century suggest adequate vitamin D_3 supplementation may decrease MS symptoms.

A 2004 study, led by Dr. Barbara M. van Amerongen of the VU Medical Center in Amsterdam, The Netherlands, concluded that consistent, optimal circulating vitamin D_3 levels may be beneficial for patients with MS. The researchers stated that optimal vitamin D_3 levels throughout the year could help to suppress MS symptoms as well as decrease MS-related complications, including increased bone fractures and muscle weakness.

In 2007, Samantha Kimball and her University of Toronto colleagues conducted a 28-week study of twelve MS patients. The results of the study indicated that daily vitamin D_3 doses of 8,000 to 10,000 IU reduced MS lesions, imaged by brain scans, by more than 50 percent!

According to a study published in a 2010 issue of *Neurology*, researchers at St. Michael's Hospital in Toronto, Canada conducted a 52-week trial of 49 (25 treatment, 24 control) MS patients with an average age of 40.5 years. Treatment patients received escalating vitamin D_3 doses and a constant daily dose of 1,200 mg of calcium. The scientists concluded that a daily vitamin D_3 dose of approximately 10,000 IU in MS patients is not only safe but effective as the MS patients "appeared to have fewer relapses" as well as "persistent reduction in T-cell proliferation compared to the study's controls. In addition, calcium levels in both trial groups were normal. In other words, a daily dose of 10,000 IU in MS patients did not endanger their calcium levels. Nonetheless, the researchers acknowledged that the classification of the evidence level obtained from the trial was insufficient to assess adequately symptomatic changes in MS patients.

Research published in the August 2012 issue of the *Annals of Neurology* indicated that higher levels of circulating vitamin D_3 are associated with fewer MS symptoms. Scientists at the University of California at San Francisco conducted a five-year study of 469 male and female MS patients to evaluate how vitamin D_3 supplementation affected disease progression. The researchers discovered that for each 10 ng/mL increase in circulating vitamin D_3, the MS patients benefited from a corresponding 15 percent decrease in new brain lesions as well as a 32 percent lower risk of inflammation of the myelin sheath.

It is important to note that when MS has been present for some years, the patient may have suffered irreversible damage to the affected nerves. Nonetheless, MS tends to progress slowly, giving promise to vitamin D_3 supplementation possibly limiting further damage. Further medical studies are essential to determine the full effectiveness of optimal vitamin D_3 levels in MS patients.

Vitamin D_3 Supplementation's Potential Value to Combat MS

The slogan of the National Multiple Sclerosis Society of America is "MS stops people from moving." I sincerely hope that adequate vitamin D_3 supplementation ultimately will prevent thousands, if not millions, of people in the world from developing MS. I also surmise MS patients with adequate vitamin

D_3 supplementation could benefit from at least a moderate alleviation of their disease's symptoms. My wish is that vitamin D_3 enables people to move! ☀

Chapter 16

Rheumatoid Arthritis

Arthritis. Many folks have seen countless commercial advertisements hawking remedies for arthritis, a disease for which there is no cure. Arthritis is the most common cause of disability in the United States, according to the Centers for Disease Control and Prevention (CDC).

Types of arthritis include rheumatoid arthritis (RA) and osteoarthritis. RA is an autoimmune disease that causes pain, swelling, and stiffness in the joints, mainly affecting the wrists, elbows, fingers, knees, ankles, toes, and neck. In addition, the immune system attacks the joint lining, causing inflammation, usually striking both sides of the body at about the same time, resulting in severely impaired mobility in the upper or lower body. Unlike the more common osteoarthritis, RA also can adversely affect the body's organ systems including the heart, lungs, kidneys, and nerves. Complications of RA can eventually destroy the joints as well as cause lung disease, heart failure, neuropathy, anemia, eye disease, or inflammation of the blood vessels.

Who is at Risk to Develop RA?

Between one and two million Americans suffer from RA. The majority of RA victims are women, though men also develop the disease. Although the debilitating illness can occur at any age, RA usually strikes persons between the ages of twenty-five and fifty.

Medical studies indicate vitamin D_3 deficiency is common among people suffering from RA.

In a 2011 issue of the *Journal of Rheumatology*, Gail S. Kerr, MD, and her colleagues assessed U.S. military veterans with RA. About 84 percent of the vitamin D_3 blood levels of 850 men, averaging sixty-four years of age, were less than 30 ng/mL, indicating low vitamin D_3 levels.

Published in 2010, a Boston University School of Public Health study revealed a greater risk of developing RA among women residing in the northeastern United States, suggesting less sunlight exposure.

A 2005 study published in the *New Zealand Medical Journal* measured the vitamin D_3 levels of fifty-five patients at a rheumatology outpatient clinic in central New Zealand. The vitamin D_3 blood levels of 78 percent of the patients were below an insufficient level of 20 ng/mL. The remaining patients' levels were severely deficient with a value less than 10 ng/mL.

How Can Vitamin D_3 Prevent RA?

Understanding how vitamin D_3 works to protect the immune system from attacking itself explains how having adequate vitamin D_3 levels could prevent RA. The Iowa Women's Health

Study conducted from 1986-97 indicated that "older women" who supplemented with vitamin D were less likely to develop RA. The research data was obtained from the subjects' self-administered questionnaires that included dietary and supplemental vitamin D intake. (The form of vitamin D was not stated in the published study.)

How Can Vitamin D₃ Treat RA?

John Hopkins University School of Medicine's Uzzma J. Haque, MD, reported on vitamin D_3 and RA research in a 2010 issue of *Clinical and Experimental Rheumatology*. The study examined sixty-two RA patients to estimate the association between their vitamin D_3 levels and disease activity, pain, and disability caused by RA. Dr. Haque concluded that vitamin D_3 deficiency was prevalent in the RA patients. Furthermore, the research revealed that RA patients with vitamin D_3 levels less than 30 ng/mL experienced more difficulty in performing basic lifestyle activities such as brushing teeth and bathing. In addition, the RA patients with a vitamin D_3 deficiency endured a higher level of tender and swollen joints as well as pain and disability.

Vitamin D₃'s Potential Value to Combat RA

Medical literature suggests that adequate vitamin D_3 supplementation may help to prevent and treat a number of autoimmune diseases. Ongoing scientific research most likely will cull additional evidence of vitamin D_3's value of protecting against RA development. Hopefully, sufficient vitamin D_3 levels also may improve symptoms of this degenerative disease. ☀

Chapter 17

Thyroid Disease

An alarming number of Americans—over 25 million—suffer from thyroid disease. Women are four times more likely than men to develop a thyroid disorder. The thyroid, a butterfly-shaped gland located in your neck, regulates your metabolism and affects every cell in your body. When your thyroid is not working properly, your body becomes unbalanced, potentially causing symptoms such as weight gain or loss and chronic fatigue as well as autoimmune disease and cancer. Let's look at how vitamin D_3 may affect thyroid health.

Thyroid Hormonal Balance

Vitamin D receptors (VDRs) are present in the cells of the pituitary, the pea-sized gland located at the base of the brain that controls your thyroid. The pituitary produces a hormone called thyroid stimulating hormone (TSH) that signals your thyroid gland to make thyroid hormone (T_3 and T_4). Thyroid hormone constantly circulates throughout your body, regulating metabolism. Either inadequate or excessive thyroid hormone can wreak havoc to your health, culminating in hypo- or hyperthyroidism. Understanding the regulating effects of VDRs in our cells, I surmise that the amount of activated vitamin D_3 in the pituitary's VDRs may be connected to the balance of thyroid hormone.

Autoimmune Thyroid Diseases

Adequate levels of vitamin D_3 may protect the immune system from attacking itself. Low vitamin D_3 levels have been linked to autoimmune thyroid diseases including Hashimoto's and Graves' thyroiditis.

Discovered one hundred years ago by a Japanese physician, Hashimoto's disease is caused by abnormal blood cells and white blood cells constantly attacking and damaging the thyroid. About 95 per cent of Hashimoto's disease patients are women. A study published in a 2011 issue of the journal *Thyroid* revealed that 92 per cent of Hashimoto's thyroiditis cases had insufficient circulating vitamin D_3 levels.

Ten times more likely to develop in women than men, Graves' disease is caused by antibodies that over stimulate thyroid hormone production, causing hyperthyroidism. Researchers who investigated Japanese female and male patients with Graves' disease over a one-year period, found a high prevalence of woefully low circulating vitamin D_3 in the female patients compared to the male subjects.

Thyroid Cancer

Incidences of thyroid cancer have doubled over the past four decades. The likelihood of women developing thyroid cancer is three times greater than for men. Activated vitamin D_3 regulates cell differentiation, cell proliferation, and cell death. If these vital functions go awry, cancer may develop. Epidemiologic studies indicate a link between vitamin D_3 and thyroid cancer. Vitamin D researcher William B. Grant, PhD, published a paper in a 2012 issue of the journal *Anticancer Research* that indicated an association between solar ultraviolet B, vitamin D_3, and cancers, including thyroid.

A relatively rare form of thyroid cancer—medullary thyroid cancer—originates in the thyroid C cells where a hormone called calcitonin is secreted. Calcitonin's functions include stimulation of vitamin D_3 production in the kidneys. The measurement of calcitonin is a diagnostic screening tool for medullary thyroid cancer. VDRs are present in the thyroid C cells. Understanding the powerful effect of activated VDRs on cell regulation, I hypothesize that activated VDRs in the C cells may possibly prevent the development of medullary thyroid cancer.

Vitamin D_3's Potential Value to Combat Thyroid disorders

Recent medical literature suggests a connection between vitamin D_3 and thyroid health. However, additional research is required to determine if thyroid dysfunction may cause vitamin D_3 deficiency or if low vitamin D_3 status may contribute to thyroid disorders. ☀

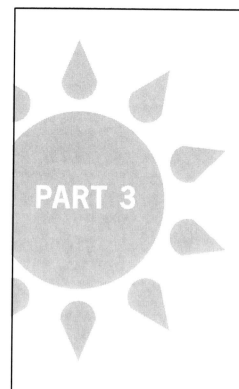

PART 3

Defending Your Life

Chapter 18

My Story, My Theory

A few years ago I began hearing positive comments about something called "vitamin D₃." I recall thinking, *I've heard of vitamin D. It is "the sunshine vitamin" and can prevent rickets. But what is vitamin D₃?*

Shortly thereafter, my husband Dave's physician insisted that he take at least 1,000 IU of vitamin D₃ daily to raise his levels. Dave and I were surprised that this vitamin was so highly touted, especially in an area with abundant sunshine.

The following month I attended my first medical lecture on vitamin D during a seminar in St. Louis. Reflecting on what I had learned at the seminar and consulting my primary care physician, I began taking 1,000 IU daily of vitamin D₃ in the soft gel form for the next several months. Six months later, my circulating vitamin D₃ was tested for the first time. The result was that my vitamin D₃ level was a shockingly low 24.4 ng/mL! I was incredulous as we had lived in Las Vegas for over a year. While I was not a sun worshipper, I certainly did not shun sunlight exposure. In fact, I welcomed it.

Intent on increasing my circulating vitamin D_3 level, my doctor prescribed 50,000 IU of "vitamin D" once a week for twelve weeks. As a vitamin D neophyte, I wholeheartedly complied with the weekly ritual of taking one oval-shaped green capsule loaded with vitamin D to improve my level. Several weeks into taking this prescription, another healthcare practitioner mentioned to me that only high-dose vitamin D_2 was available by prescription. She suggested I double-check the prescription information. Sure enough, I was taking vitamin D_2, a less effective form of vitamin D! Consequently, I expressed my concern to my doctor; immediately stopped taking the vitamin D_2 prescription; and doubled my daily vitamin D_3 soft gel intake to 2,000 IU.

Three months later, my circulating vitamin D_3 level had only increased to 33.6 ng/mL, still well below my doctor's minimal goal of 50 ng/mL. Clearly, I was taking either inadequate amounts of vitamin D_3 or the soft gel supplement was not well-absorbed by my body. At my doctor's suggestion, I commenced taking vitamin D_3 drops sublingually, or under the tongue.

What is the Optimal Circulating Vitamin D_3 Level?

While attempting to raise my circulating vitamin D_3 level, I asked myself, *How much circulating vitamin D_3 is absorbed by the cells?* My information may surprise you.

Opinions concerning the optimal circulating vitamin D_3 level differ greatly. The majority of the global medical community perceived circulating vitamin D_3 levels greater than 100 ng/

mL to be high. At the time of this writing, I am unaware of agreement about the optimal range of circulating vitamin D_3. I also think the optimal range may differ according to one's age, skin color, and body fat, factors that affect vitamin D_3 production.

Circulating vitamin D_3 must bind to vitamin D_3 receptors before it becomes activated, indicating a direct correlation between circulating vitamin D_3 and activated vitamin D_3—the D_3 that resides and, in some cases, is produced, in our cells. If measured activated vitamin D_3 is less than 100 percent in the body, the circulating vitamin D_3 level can be safely increased by obtaining initial vitamin D_3 from UVB light, diet, or supplementation.

My Case Study: Vitamin D_3 Testing

Given my understanding of circulating vitamin D_3 levels, I used myself as a "guinea pig" to test my theory by undergoing routine vitamin D and micronutrient tests.

In June 2010 and 2011, I underwent concurrent blood draws submitted for two separate evaluations: the standard 25(OH) vitamin D test and a micronutrient (including vitamin D_3) analysis of my white blood cells. LabCorp, Inc. evaluated my circulating vitamin D_3 level. SpectraCell Laboratories, Inc. conducted the micronutrient testing.

My circulating vitamin D_3 level in June 2010 was 137 ng/ mL—a value that many medical professionals consider excessive. However, my micronutrient—or cellular—test revealed only sufficient amounts of activated vitamin D_3, but not "over the top." The SpectraCell score was 67 percent, indicating that the vitamin D_3 in my cells was above the "greater than 50 percent reference range" for female and male patients age twelve or older. One year later, the standard blood and cellular tests revealed a similar correlation. In my opinion, the laboratory data suggest:

I can safely increase my intake of vitamin D_3 according to the percentage difference between my activated vitamin D_3 levels and 100. (Subtract micronutrient value from 100 percent. In my case I could increase my daily dose by 33 percent.)[5]

The optimal circulating vitamin D_3 level, at least for me, is about 180 ng/mL. To date, my highest circulating vitamin D_3 level has been 194.7 ng/mL. Because this number was significantly out of the current range, the laboratory noted that the value had been "verified by repeat analysis." I primarily attribute this astounding increase to being kissed (without sunscreen) by the Polynesian sun for a week during optimal weather conditions only days prior to the blood test. In general, my circulating vitamin D_3 level has hovered around 100 ng/mL during the past two years.

My Theory

Until the medical community reaches agreement on an optimal circulating vitamin D_3 level, I think the most effective

---

[5] The VDRs in my cells can accommodate additional activated vitamin D_3 equivalent to the result of a couple calculations involving both the circulating and activated vitamin D_3 levels. (Circulating = 137 ng/mL; activated = 67 percent. Divide 137 by the remaining percentage, 33, to obtain 46 ng/mL. Add 46 to 137 = 183 ng/mL.)

method for understanding true vitamin D_3 status in individuals is by conducting intracellular micronutrient testing. Why? The results of a blood serum test only analyze a "snapshot" or one-moment-in-time, i.e., when the blood was collected, of one's vitamin D_3 level (and other evaluated nutrients). Conversely, intracellular testing reveals the short-term history of an individual's functional nutritional status. When thinking about my health, I prefer to understand my cells' history than simply view a glimpse of nutritional status in my bloodstream during one moment.

The bottom line of one's health is the state of one's cellular function. Based on the anecdotal evidence stated above, I theorize that the optimal vitamin D_3 range should be increased to reflect how much activated vitamin D_3 can be accommodates in our cells. If my hypothesis is correct, daily vitamin D_3 supplementation could be safely increased to at least 10,000 IU.[6] As scientific research on vitamin D_3 continues, I surmise that the optimal circulating vitamin D_3 level could eventually approach 200 ng/mL.

In the final chapter you will understand how easily, safely, and inexpensively you can use vitamin D_3 to "Defend Your Life." ☀

---

[6] I also believe that the medical community should consider factors such as age, body fat, and skin pigmentation when developing updated reference values for circulating vitamin D_3.

Chapter 19

Defend Your Life

To say vitamin D has anti-inflammatory, antimicrobial, antiviral, anti-anything properties is an understatement. Vitamin D may be one of our most reliable proactive ingredients in bolstering comprehensive immunity and reinforcing the body's natural defenses.
—Michael Holick, PhD, MD.

Now that you have almost finished reading this book, you know how vitamin D_3 can "defend your life" by understanding that having adequate vitamin D_3 in your cells may:

- Reduce the risk of developing cancer.

- Prevent autoimmune diseases including multiple sclerosis and rheumatoid arthritis.

- Avoid contracting viral infections including the common cold and influenza.

- Prevent and treat dental health issues.

- Lower the risk of children developing autism.

- Decrease the likelihood of cardiovascular disease.

- Enhance athletic performance.

- Prevent and treat thyroid disorders.

- Influence biological age.

Pretty impressive benefits, huh? By implementing a simple plan to take vitamin D_3 daily and periodically monitoring your results, you can enjoy improved quality of life by being healthier as well as more productive.

In honor of the 2012 London Olympics, I offer a winning approach that can make vitamin D_3 a part of your personal life's Olympics and afford you a healthier and longer life!

BRONZE MEDAL

☐ Take at least 2,000 to 5,000 IU of vitamin D_3 supplements daily.

SILVER MEDAL

☐ Take at least 2,000 to 5,000 IU of vitamin D_3 supplements daily.

☐ After three months, take a blood test to ascertain your vitamin D_3 level. Adjust your daily intake of vitamin D_3 supplementation according to blood test results.

~~~~~~

GOLD MEDAL

☐ Take at least 2,000 to 5,000 IU of vitamin D_3 supplements daily.

☐ After three months, take a blood test to ascertain your vitamin D_3 level. Adjust your daily intake of vitamin D_3 supplementation according to blood test results.

☐ After six months, take a micronutrient intracellular test (e.g., SpectraCell) to determine how much activated vitamin D_3 is in your cells. Continue taking vitamin D_3 supplements and monitor your vitamin D_3 in concert with your healthcare practitioner.

~~~~~~

What Type of Vitamin D_3 Supplement Should I Take?

First and foremost, please ensure that the supplement you choose is vitamin D_3 (*three*) containing cholecalciferol. If the supplement label only states "vitamin D," beware.

Vitamin D_3 is fat-soluble so the best-absorbed supplements are oil-based and in the forms of liquid soft gels and drops. These easy-to-swallow supplements are readily available over the counter and online. (Forget those huge, cheap bottles of vitamin D tablets that are available at discounted "big box" stores; you would be wasting your time, money, and health.)

The best time to take your vitamin D_3 supplement is during or immediately after your fattiest meal of the day. Place your vitamin D_3 supplements in a cool, dry location where you will remember to take them daily.

How Do I Get Tested for Circulating (blood) Vitamin D₃?

Undergoing a blood test to learn your circulating vitamin D_3 level is easy. You can get the test called 25-hydroxyvitamin D or 25(OH)D from your healthcare practitioner. Routine blood work often includes a vitamin D_3 evaluation but I recommend double-checking with your practitioner before your blood is drawn to ensure that the vitamin D_3 test is included on the laboratory order form. Many healthcare plans cover all, or at least partial, costs of the blood test. (The ICD-9 code is 268.9.) In addition, blood screening kits for 25(OH)D are available online from reputable companies. See "Additional Resources" for some U.S. laboratories that perform 25(OH)D blood serum testing.

How Do I Get Tested for Activated (cellular) Vitamin D₃?

Taking a cellular test to learn your activated vitamin D_3 level is also simple. Request a blood draw from a participating doctor or a laboratory stated on the SpectraCell[7] website: www. spectracell.com. No overnight fasting is usually required. Your doctor's office or a SpectraCell-approved facility draws two tubes of blood that are sent to the lab. SpectraCell analyzes the nutritional history of your white blood cells. Within two to three weeks, you and your clinician receive a detailed report that explains your cellular health by specifying the level of thirty-

[7] Please note that the author and Smilin Sue Publishing, LLC have neither a financial nor a personal association with this entity. This corporation is the sole laboratory with which the author is familiar to evaluate intracellular nutrient testing.

four individual vitamins, minerals, amino acids, metabolites, antioxidants as well as carbohydrate metabolism indicators. The easy-to-understand report includes color graphs of each micronutrient and explains how to correct any deficiencies. Within the context of this book, the great news is that the report allows you to understand the amount of vitamin D_3 that has been stored in your cells! (See "Micronutrient Testing" for further information.)

According to SpectraCell's public information, the Micronutrient Testing is "a next generation blood test for measuring specific vitamins, minerals, antioxidants, and other essential micronutrients within an individual's white blood cells ... it is the gold standard for this type of test." On the one hand, I agree that this test is the "gold standard" for reasons mentioned in this chapter. On the other hand, I take issue that Micronutrient Testing is "a next generation blood test." This test is for today! Remember, your quality of life depends upon the state of your body's cells. If you have the resources to undergo this test every year or so, I encourage you to do so.

Empower Your Health with Vitamin D_3

In this book I have explained vitamin D_3 including how it has helped many people by preventing a wide array of diseases and by treating some medical conditions. The scientific future holds more promising evidence of vitamin D_3's benefits. I sincerely hope you, your family, and friends experience an improved quality of life from acquiring vitamin D_3 from supplements, sunlight, and diet. The map to better health is in your hands. Now is the time to follow the path to better living. ☀

Additional Resources

I encourage you to empower yourself by learning as much as you can about the fascinating world of vitamin D_3.

Books

The Athlete's Edge Faster, Quicker, Stronger with Vitamin D, John Cannell, MD, Here & Now Books, 2011.

The Sunlight Solution, Laurie Winn Carlson, Promethus Books, 2009.

The Vitamin D Cure, James E. Dowd, MD and Diane Stafford, John Wiley & Sons, Inc., 2008.

The Vitamin D Solution, Michael Holick, PhD, MD, Hudson Street Press, 2010.

The Vitamin D Revolution, Soram Khalsa, MD, Hay House, Inc., 2009.

Vitamin K_2 and the Calcium Paradox, Kate Rheaume-Bleue, ND, John Wiley & Sons Canada, Ltd., 2012.

African-American Healthy, Richard W. Walker, Jr., MD, Square One Publishers, Inc., 2011.

Non-profit Vitamin D Organizations

www.grassrootshealth.net. Carole Baggerly, Director, GrassrootsHealth, has launched an international public health campaign to solve vitamin D deficiency by focusing on testing and education.

www.vitamindcouncil.org. Founded by John J. Cannell, MD, the Vitamin D Council's mission is "to educate the general public and health professionals on vitamin D, sun exposure, and the vitamin D deficiency pandemic."

Circulating Vitamin D₃ Testing

Labrix Clinical Services. www.labrix.com. Telephone: 1-877-656-9596.

Life Extension Foundation. www.lef.org/blood. Telephone: 1-800-208-3444.

ZRT Labs. www.zrtlab.com. Telephone: 1-866-600-1636.

Conversion Tables

To clarify measurements of vitamin D₃ dosages, doses, and circulating levels, conversion tables are provided:

Vitamin D₃ Supplementation		
40 IU	=	1 mcg
400 IU	=	10 mcg
1,000 IU	=	25 mcg
2,000 IU	=	50 mcg
5,000 IU	=	125 mcg
50,000 IU	=	1,250 mcg or 1.25 mg

Circulating Vitamin D₃ Levels**		
1 ng/mL	=	2.5 nmol/L
30 ng/mL	=	75 nmol/L
50 ng/mL	=	125 nmol/L
100 ng/mL	=	250 nmol/L

Note: The number "2.5" is the key to converting reference values for circulating vitamin D₃ levels. Simply multiply the ng/mL value by 2.5 to obtain the nmol/L value, or divide the nmol/L value by 2.5 to ascertain the value expressed in ng/mL.

Micronutrient Cellular Testing

SpectraCell Laboratories' Micronutrient Cellular Test (www.spectracell.com) includes readings for activated vitamin

D_3 as well as values for thirty-three other vitamins, minerals, amino acids, etc. that are stored in your cells. The test results present a history of the nutrients in the cells over the past several months.

A major benefit of micronutrient testing is the capability to understand and treat, if necessary, the vitamin D_3 levels in your cells—where it really counts for health. You can obtain cellular testing for Vitamin D_3 levels (as well as many other cellular components) through SpectraCell Laboratories, Inc. SpectraCell was established in Houston, Texas in 1983, and owns a patented technology that analyzes over thirty essential vitamins, minerals, and other nutrient functions within one's vast number of cells.

The laboratory assesses the history of one's nutritional intake by evaluating vitamins, minerals, and other necessary micronutrients, including antioxidants, in white blood cells (WBCs), or lymphocytes. Easily isolated from other whole blood cells, most WBCs collected during a blood draw are in a state of rest and live for about four to six months. (Hence, the tested WBCs characterize a history of one's nutrient status.) SpectraCell develops the extracted cells in a specific culture medium that contains optimal levels of the essential nutrients being tested. Mitogens—chemical substances that are usually proteins—are added to promote the division and growth stimulation of resting cells. SpectraCell measures the cellular growth rate by DNA synthesis and the available amount of each nutrient to assess the nutrient status over the cultured cells' resting lifespan.

Is this testing expensive? The cost of SpectraCell's Micro-nutrient Test is surprisingly reasonable. Many health insurance plans cover at least part of this medical evaluation. When applicable, insured patients are responsible for co-payments and/or deductible costs. In June 2011, I paid an insurance co-payment of $170 to obtain SpectraCell analysis of my intracellular health, including activated vitamin D_3 status. Over a year's time, the cost of this test—at least in my case—equates to about 47 U.S. cents a day. ☀

Index

L
Lanolin   34
Lappe, Joan M.   66
Latitude   23, 77, 89, 117, 121
Life Extension Foundation   150
Lucas, Robyn M.   121
Lupus   48, 107

M
Magliato, Kathy   82
Magnesium   39, 42–43
Melanin   24
Menaquinone   40–41
Mongolia   88
Multiple sclerosis   16, 20–21, 48, 106–107, 115–116, 119, 121, 124, 143
Munger, Kassandra L.   118–119
Muscle strength   55, 84
Myelin sheath   116, 120, 124

N
Natto   41
Netherlands, The   119, 123
New Zealand   37, 89, 115, 121, 128
Nieves, Jeri   117
Nurses' Health Study   118

O
Obesity. *See* Weight
Olympics   144
Osteoarthritis. *See* Arthritis
Osteoporosis   27, 41, 43, 48

P

Pancreas 98–100
    beta islet cells 98–99, 102–103
Phlebitis 81, 84
Phylloquinone 40
Pituitary 131–132
Pregnancy 48, 57, 59–61, 95, 99–100, 117–118
    newborns 60, 95
Prostate cancer 76–79

Q

Quality of life 17, 19, 33, 58, 71, 90, 144, 147, 177

R

Ramagopalan, Sreeram 120
Randomized controlled trial (RCT) 36–37, 66, 85, 88, 92, 94, 102, 111–112
Rheumatoid arthritis. *See* Arthritis
Rickets 27, 34, 99, 137

S

Sarcoidosis 31
Scotland 117
Scragg, Robert 82
Spain 75, 78
SpectraCell Laboratories 139–140, 145–147, 150–152
SPF. *See* Sunscreen
Sports 51–55
Stanley Cup 52
Stroke 81, 83–84
Sunbathing 21
Sunblock. *See* Sunscreen

Vitamin A   25, 39–40, 43

Vitamin D_3 supplementation   25, 31, 43, 51–53, 55, 60–63,
    69, 72, 75, 79, 85, 88, 90–91, 93, 95, 98–99, 103, 111–
    112, 118, 120–124, 129, 141, 144–145

Vitamin D_3 supplements   20, 25–26, 30–31, 34, 37, 52–53,
    60, 62–63, 112, 119, 144–146

Vitamin D_1 33

Vitamin D_2 20, 25, 33–38, 138

Vitamin D_4 33

Vitamin D_5 33

Vitamin D Council   52, 60–62, 99, 111, 149, 177

Vitamin D forms   33–34

Vitamin D receptors (VDR)   29–30, 59, 68, 70–71, 73, 75,
    77–79, 83, 98–99, 106, 131–133, 140

Vitamin K_1 40

Vitamin K_2 39–43, 84, 149

W

Weight   23, 82, 100–101, 103, 131

Z

Zaidi, Sarfraz   92–93

Bibliography

Amano Y, Komiyama K, Makishima M. "Vitamin D and periodontal disease." *J Oral Sci.* 2009 Mar; 51(1):11-20.

Armas LA, Hollis BW, Heaney RP. "Vitamin D_2 is much less effective than vitamin D_3 in humans." *J Clin Endrocrinol Metab.* 2004 Nov;89(11):5387-91.

Anderson JL, May HT, Horne BD, Bair TL, Hall NL, Carlquist JF, Lappe DL, Muhlestein JB, Intermountain Heart Collaborative (IHC) Study Group. "Relation of vitamin D deficiency to cardiovascular risk factors, disease status, and incident events in a general healthcare population." *Am J Cardiol.* 2010 Oct 1;106(7):963-8. Epub 2010 Aug 11.

Asp K. "Running on D: The 'sun vitamin' may boost performance, but you probably aren't getting enough." *Runner's World*, December 2009.

Bartley, J. "Vitamin D, innate immunity and upper respiratory tract infection." *J Laryngol Otol.* 2010 May;124(5):465-9. Epub 2010 Jan 13.

Boggess KA, Espinola JA, Moss K, Beck J, Offenbacher S, Camargo CA. "Vitamin D Status and Periodontal Disease among Pregnant Women." *J Periodontol.* 2011 Feb;82(2):195-200. Epub 2010 Sep 1.

Bortman P, Folgueira MA, Katayama ML, Snitcovsky IM, Brentani MM. "Antiproliferative effects of 1,25-dihydroxyvitamin D_3 on breast cells: a mini review." *Braz J Med Biol Res.* 2002 Jan;35(1):1-9.

Boyle CA, Boulet S, Schieve LA, Cohen RA, Blumberg SJ, Yeargin-Allsopp M, Visser S, Kogan MD. "Trends in the Prevalence of Developmental Disabilities in US Children, 1997-2008." *Pediatrics.* 2011 Jun;127(6):1034-42. Epub 2011 May 23.

Burton JM, Kimball S, Vieth R, Bar-Or A, Dosch HM, Cheung R, Gagne D, D'Souza C, Ursell M, O'Connor P. "A Phase I/II Dose-Escalation Trial of Vitamin D₃ and Calcium in Multiple Sclerosis." *Neurology.* 2010 June 8; 74(23):1852-9.

Byers SW, Rowlands T, Beildeck M, Bong YS. "Mechanism of action of vitamin D and receptor in colorectal cancer prevention and treatment." *Rev Endocr Metab Disord.* 2012 Mar;13(1):31-8.

Camargo CA Jr, Ganmaa D, Frazier AL, Kirchberg FF, Stuart JJ, Kleinman K, Sumberzul N, Rich-Edwards JW. "Randomized trial of vitamin D supplementation and risk of acute respiratory tract infection in Mongolia." *Pediatrics.* 2012 Sep;130(3)e561-7. doi:10.1542/peds.2011-3029. Epub 2012 Aug 20.

Camargo CA Jr, Ingham T, Wickens K, Thadhani RI, Silvers KM, Epton MJ, Town GI, Espinola JA, Crane J; New Zealand Asthma and Allergy Cohort Study Group. "Vitamin D status of newborns in New Zealand." *Br J Nutr.* 2010 Oct;104(7):1051-7. Epub 2010 Apr 29.

Cannell, John. *The Athlete's Edge Faster Quicker Stronger with Vitamin D.* Here & Now Books. 2011.

Cannell JJ. "Autism and vitamin D." *Med Hypotheses.* 2008;70(4):750-9. Epub 2007 Oct 24.

Cannell JJ. "On the aetiology of autism." *Acta Paediatr.* 2010 August; 99(8): 1128-1130.

Cannell JJ. "Peak Athletic Performance and Vitamin D." *Vitamin D Council Newsletter.* March 2007.

Cannell JJ, Hollis BW, Sorenson MB, Taft TN, Anderson JJ. "Athletic performance and vitamin D." *Med Sci Sports Exerc.* 2009 May;41(5):1102-10.

Cannell JJ, Hollis BW, Zasloff M, Heaney RP. "Diagnosis and treatment of vitamin D deficiency." *Expert Opin Pharmacother.* 2008;9(1):107-18.

Cannell JJ, Vieth R, Umhau JC, Holick MF, Grant WB, Madronich S, Garland CF, Giovannucci E. "Epidemic influenza and vitamin D." *Epidemiol Infect.* 2006 Dec;134(6):1129-40. Epub 2006 Sep 7.

Cannell JJ, Zasloff M, Garland CF, Scragg R, Giovannucci E. "On the epidemiology of influenza." *Vir J.* 2008 Feb 25;5:29.

Carlson, Laurie Winn. *The Sunlight Solution: Why More Sun Exposure and Vitamin D Are Essential to Your Health.* Prometheus Books. 2009.

Chen TC, Holick MF. "Vitamin D and prostate cancer prevention and treatment." *Trends Endocrinol Metab.* 2003 Nov;14(9):423-30.

Chlebowski RT, et al, and Women's Health Initiative Investigators. "Calcium plus vitamin D supplementation and the risk of breast cancer." *J Natl Cancer Inst.* 2008 Nov 19;100(22):1562-4 and *J Natl Cancer Inst.* 2009 May 6;101(9):690; author reply 690-1.

Chui G. "Vitamin D deficiency among patients attending a central New Zealand rheumatology outpatient clinic." *NZ Med J.* 2005 Nov 11;188(1225):U1727.

Close GL, Russell J, Cobley JN, Owens DJ, Wilson G, Gregson W, Fraser WD, Morton JP. "Assessment of vitamin D concentration in non-supplemented professional athletes and healthy adults during the winter months in the UK: implications for skeletal muscle function." *J Sports Sci.* Epub 2012 Oct 22.

Crew KD, Gammon MD, Steck SE, Hershman DL, Cremers S, Dwora-kowski E, Shane E, Terry MB, Desai M, Teitelbaum SL, Neugut AI, Santella RM. "Association between plasma 25-hydroxyvitaminD and breast cancer risk." *Cancer Prev Res* (Phila). 2009 Jun;2(6):598-604. Epub 2009 May 26.

Cuomo, Margaret I., *A World Without Cancer.* Rodale Inc. 2012.

Dietrich T, Joshipura KJ, Dawson-Hughes B, Bischoff-Ferrari HA. "Association between serum concentrations of 25-hydroxyvitamin D₃ and periodontal disease in US Population." *Am J Clin Nutr.* 2004 Jul;80(1):103-13.

Dietrich T, Nunn M, Dawson-Hughes B, Biscoff-Ferrari HA. "Association between serum concentrations of 25-hydroxyvitamin D and gingival inflammation." *Am J Clin Nutr.* 2005 Sep;82(3):575-80.

Dobson R, Giovannoni G, Ramagopalan D. "The month of birth effect in multiple sclerosis: systematic review, meta-analysis and effect of latitude." *J Neurol Neurosurg Psychiatry.* Epub 2012 Nov 14.

Dowd, James E. and Diane Stafford. *The Vitamin D Cure.* John Wiley & Sons, Inc. 2008.

Edich RF, Mason SS, Dahlstrom JJ, Swainston E, Long WB 3rd, Gubler K. "Pandemic preparedness for swine flu influenza in the United States." *J Environ Pathol Toxicol Oncol.* 2009;28(4):261-4.

Embry AF, Snowdon LR, Vieth R. "Vitamin D and seasonal fluctuations of gadolinium-enhancing magnetic resonance imaging lesions in multiple sclerosis." *Ann Neurol.* 2000 Aug;48(2):271-2.

Faloon, William. *Pharmocracy.* Praktikos Books. 2011.

Feldman D, Pike JW, Adams JS. *Vitamin D* (Third Edition), Volumes I and II. Academic Press. 2011.

Fossel M, Blackburn G, and Woynarowski D. *The Immortality Edge.* John Wiley & Sons, Inc. 2011.

Gagnon C, Lu ZX, Magliano DJ, Dunstan DW, Shaw JE, Zimmet PZ, Sikaris K, Grantham N, Ebeling PR, Daly RM. "Serum 25-hydroxyvitamin D, calcium intake, and risk of type 2 diabetes after 5 years: results from a national population-based prospective study." *Diabetes Care.* 2011 May;34(5):1133-8. Epub 2011 Mar 23.

Ganji V, Zhang X, Shaikh N, Tangricha V. "Serum 25-hydroxyvitamin D concentrations are associated with prevalence of metabolic syndrome and various cardiometabolic risk factors in US children and adolescents based on assay-adjusted serum 25-hydroxyvitamin D data from NHANES 2001-2006." *Am J Clin Nutr.* 2011 Jul;94(1):225-33. Epub 2011 May 25.

Garcia MN, Hildebolt CF, Miley DD, Dixon DA, Couture RA, Anderson Spearie CL, Langenwalter EM, Shannon WD, Deych E, Mueller C, Civitelli R. "One-year Effects of Vitamin D and Calcium Supplementation on Chronic Periodontitis." *J Periodontol.* 2011 Jan:82(1):25-32.

Garland CF, French CB, Baggerly LL, Heaney RP. "Vitamin D Supplement Doses and Serum 25-Hydroxyvitamin D in the Range Associated with Cancer Prevention." *J Anticancer Research.* 2011 Feb;31(2):607-611.

Garland CF, Garland FC. "Do sunlight and vitamin D reduce the likelihood of colon cancer?" *Int J Epidemiol.* 1980 Sep;9(3):227-31.

Garland CF, Gorham ED, Mohr SB, Garland FC. "Vitamin D for cancer prevention: global perspective." *Ann Epidemiol.* 2009 Jul;19(7):468-83.

Garland CF, Gorham ED, Mohr SB, Grant WB, Giovannucci EL, Lipkin M, Newmark H, Holick MF, Garland FC. "Vitamin D and prevention of breast cancer: pooled analysis." *J Steroid Biochem Mol Biol.* 2007 Mar;103(3-5):708-11.

Garland FC, Garland, CF, Gorham ED, Young, JF. "Geographic variation in breast cancer mortality in the United States: a hypothesis involving exposure to solar radiation." *Preventive Medicine* 1990 Nov;19(6):614-22.

Ginde AA, Mansbach JM, Camargo, Jr. CA. "Association between serum 25-hydroxyvitamin D level and upper respiratory tract infection in the third National Health and Nutrition Survey." *Arch InternMed.* 2009 Feb 23;169(4):384-90.

Giovannucci E., "Epidemiology of vitamin D and colorectal cancer: casual or causal link?" *J Steroid Biochem Mol Biol.* 2010 Jul;121(1-2):349-54. Epub 2010 Apr 14.

Gorham ED, Garland CF, Garland FC, Grant WB, Mohr SB, Lipkin M, Newmark HL, Giovannucci E, Wei M, Holick MF. "Vitamin D and prevention of colorectal cancer." *J Steroid Biochem Mol Biol.* 2005 Oct;97(1-2):179-94. Epub 2005 Oct 19.

Gorham ED, Garland FC, Garland CF. "Sunlight and breast cancer incidence in the USSR." *Intl J Epid.* 1990;19(4):820-4.

Grant WB. "Ecological studies of the UVB-vitamin D-cancer hypothesis." *Anticancer Res.* 2012 Jan;32(1):223-36.

Grant WB, Boucher BJ. "Requirements for Vitamin D across the Life Span." *Biol Res Nurs.* 2011 Jan 17.

Handel AE, Jarvis L, McLaughlin R, Fries A, Ebers GC, Ramagoplan SV. "The Epidemiology of Multiple Sclerosis in Scotland: Inferences from Hospital Admissions." *PLoS One.* 2011 Jan 27;6(1):e14606.

Handunnetthi L, Ramagopalan SV, Ebers GC. "Multiple sclerosis, vitamin D, and HLA-DRB1*15. *Neurology.* 2010 Jan 8;74(23):1905-10.

Haque UJ, Bartlett SJ. "Relationships among vitamin D, disease activity, pain and disability in rheumatoid arthritis." *Clin Exp Rheumatol.* 2010 Sep-Oct;28(5):745-7. Epub 2010 Oct 22.

Harris S. "Emerging roles of vitamin D: More reasons to address widespread vitamin D insufficiency." *Mol Aspects Med.* 2008 Dec;29(6):359-60.

Heaney RP, Recker RR, Grote J, Horst RL, Armas LA. "Vitamin D_3 is more potent than vitamin D_2 in humans." *J Clin Endocrinol Metab.* 2011 Mar;96(3):E447-52. Epub 2010 Dec 22.

Hendrickson WK, Flavin R, Kasperzyk JL, Fiorentino M, Fang F, Lis R, Fiore C, Penney KL, Ma J, Kantoff PW, Stampfer MJ, Loda M, Mucci LA, Giovannucci E. "Vitamin D receptor protein expression in tumor tissue and prostate cancer progression." *J Clin Oncol.* 2011 Jun 10;29(17):2378-85. Epub 2011 May 2.

Hines SL, Jorn HK, Thompson KM, Larson JM. "Breast cancer survivors and vitamin D: a review." *Nutrition.* 2010 Mar;26(3):255-62. Epub 2009 Dec 8.

Holick MF. "Environmental factors that influence the cutaneous production of vitamin D." *Am J Clin Nutr.* 1995 Mar;61(3 Suppl):638S-645S.

Holick MF, Biancuzzo RM, Chen TC, Klein EK, Young A, Bibuld D, Reitz R, Salameh W, Ameri A, Tannenbaum AD. "Vitamin D_2 is as effective as vitamin D_3 in maintaining circulating concentrations of 25-hydroxyvitamin D." *J Clin Endocrin Metab.* 2008 March; 93(3): 677-81.

Holick, Michael F. *The Vitamin D Solution.* Hudson Street Press. 2010.

Holick MF. McCollum award lecture, 1994: "Vitamin D – new horizons for the 21st century." *Am J Clin Nutr.* 1994 Oct;60(4):619-30.

Holmoy T. "Vitamin D status modulates the immune response to Epstein Barr virus: Synergistic effect of risk factors in multiple sclerosis." *Med Hypotheses.* 2008:70(1):66-9. Epub 2007 Jun 14.

Houghton LA, Vieth R. "The case against ergocalciferol (vitamin D_2) as a vitamin supplement." *Am J Clin Nutr.* 2006 Oct;84(4):694-7.

Hypponen E, Laara E, Reunanen A, Jarvelin MR, Virtanen SM. "Intake of vitamin D and risk of type 1 diabetes: a birth-cohort study." *Lancet.* 2001 Nov3;358(9292):1500-3.

Keebler, Craig A. *Know Your D. Optimizing Your Health with Vitamin D.* SCBM, PLLC. 2010.

Kerr GS, Sabahi I, Richards JS, Caplan L, Cannon GW, Reimold A, Thiele GM, Johnson D, Mikuls TR. "Prevalence of vitamin D insufficiency/deficiency in rheumatoid arthritis and associations with disease severity and activity." *J Rheumatol*. 2011 Jan;38(1):53-9. Epub 2010 Oct 15.

Khalsa, Soram. *The Vitamin D Revolution*. Hay House, Inc. 2009.

Khare D, Godbole NM, Pawar SD, Mohan V, Pandey G, Gupta S, Kumar D, Dhole TN, Godbole MM. "Calcitriol [1,25[OH]2 D_3] pre- and post-treatment suppresses inflammatory response to influenza A (H1N1) infection in human lung A549 epithelial cells." *Eur J Nutr*. 2012 Sep 27.

Khoo AL, Chai L, Koenen H, Joosten I, Netea M, van der Van A. "Translating the role of vitamin D_3 in infectious diseases." *Crit Rev Microbiol*. 2012 May;38(2):122-35. Epub 2012 Feb 5.

Kimball SM, Ursell MR, O'Connor P, Vieth R. "Safety of vitamin D_3 in adults with multiple sclerosis." *Am J Clin Nutr*. 2007 Sep;86(3):645-51.

Kivity S, Agmon-Levin N, Zisappl M, Shapira Y, Nagy EV, Danko K, Szekanecz Z, Langevitz P, Shoenfeld Y. "Vitamin D and autoimmune thyroid diseases." *Cell Mol Immunol*. 2011 May;8(3):243-7. Epub 2011 Jan 31.

Kragt J, van Amerongen B, Killestein J, Dijkstra C, Uitdehaag B, Polman Ch, Lips P. "Higher levels of 25-hydroxyvitamin D are associated with a lower incidence of multiple sclerosis only in women." *Mult Scler*. 2009 Jan;15(1):9-15. Epub 2008 Aug 13.

Krall EA, Garcia RI, Dawson-Hughes B. "Increased risk of tooth loss is related to bone loss at the whole body, hip, and spine." *Calcif Tissue Int*. 1996 Dec;59(6):433-7.

Krall EA, Wehler C, Garcia RI, Harris SS, Dawson-Hughes B. "Calcium and vitamin D supplements reduce tooth loss in the elderly." *Am J Med*. 2001 Oct 15;111(6):452-6.

Krishnan AV, Feldman D. "Mechanisms of the anti-cancer and anti-inflammatory actions of vitamin D." *Annu Rev Pharmacol Toxicol.*, 2011 Feb 10;51:311-36.

Lappe JM, Travers-Gustafson D, Davies KM, Recker RR, Heaney RP. "Vitamin D and calcium supplementation cancer risk: results of a randomized trial." *Am J Clin Nutr.* 2007 Jun;85(6):1586-91.

Larriba MJ, Ordonez-Moran P, Chicote I, Martin-Fernandez G, Puig I, Munoz A, Palmer HG. "Vitamin D receptor deficiency enhances Wnt/beta-catenin signaling and tumor burden in colon cancer." *PLoS One.* 2011;6(8):e23524. Epub 2011 Aug 15.

Lindqvist PG, Epstein E, Olsson H. "Does an active sun exposure lower the risk of venous thrombotic events? A D-lightful hypothesis." *J Thromb Haemost.* 2009 Apr;7(4):605-10.

Lloyd-Jones D, Adams RJ, Brown TM, et al. "Heart Disease and Stroke Statistics—2010 Update. A Report from the American Heart Association Statistics Committee and Stroke Statistics Subcommittee." *Circulation.* 2010;121:e1-e170.

Logan VF, Gray AR, Peddie MC, Harper MJ, Houghton LA. "Long-term vitamin D_3 supplementation is more effective than vitamin D_2 in maintaining serum 25-hydroxyvitamin D status over the winter months." *Br J Nutr.* 2012 Jul 11; 1-7.

Loke TW, Sevfi D, Khadra M. "Prostate cancer incidence in Australia correlates inversely with solar radiation." *BJU Int.* 2011 Nov;108 Suppl 2:66-70.

Lucas RM, Ponsonby AL, Dear K, Valery PC, Pender MP, Taylor BV, Kilpatrick TJ, Dwyer T, Chapman C, va der Mei I, Williams D, McMichael AJ. "Sun exposure and vitamin D are independent risk factors for CNS demyelination." *Neurology.* 2011 Feb 8;76(6):540-8.

MacLaughlin J, Holick MF. "Aging decreases the capacity of human skin to produce vitamin D₃." *J Clin Invest.* 1985 Oct;76(4):1536-8.

Madrid, Eric. *Vitamin D Prescription.* www.booksurge.com. 2009.

Merlino LA, Curtis J, Mikulis TR, Cerhan JR, Criswell LA, Saag KG. "Iowa Women's Health Study. Vitamin D intake is inversely associated with rheumatoid arthritis: results from the Iowa Women's Health Study." *Arthritis & Rheumatism.* 2004 Jan;50(1):72-7.

Merrill, Michael D. *Vitamin D: Antidote to Winter and the Darkness.* Lulu.com. 2006.

Mitri J, Dawson-Hughes B, Hu FB, Pittas AG. "Effects of vitamin D and calcium supplementation on pancreatic {beta} cell function, insulin sensitivity, and glycemia in adults at high risk of diabetes: the Calcium and Vitamin D for Diabetes Mellitus (CaDDM) randomized controlled trial." *Am J Clin Nutr.* 2011 Aug;94(2):486-94. Epub 2011 Jun 29.

Mitri J, Muraru MD, Pittas AG. "Vitamin D and type 2 diabetes: a systematic review." *Eur J Clin Nutr.* 2011 Sep;65(9):1005-15. Epub 2011 Jul 6.

Mohr SB, Gorham ED, Alcaraz JE, Kane CI, Macera CA, Parsons JK, Wingard DL, Garland CF. "Serum 25-hydroxyvitamin D and prevention of breast cancer: pooled analysis." *Anticancer Res.* 2011 Sep;31(9):2939-48.

Mohr SB, Gorham ED, Alcaraz JE, Kane CI, Macera CA, Parsons JK, Wingard DL, Garland CF. "Does the evidence for an inverse relationship between serum vitamin D status and breast cancer risk satisfy the Hill criteria?" *Dermatoendocrinol.* 2012 Apr 1;4(2):152-7.

Morton JP, Iqbal Z, Drust B, Burgess D, Close GL, Brukner PD. "Seasonal variation in vitamin D status in professional soccer players of the English Premier League." *Appl Physiol Nutr Metab.* 2012 Aug;37(4):798-802. Epub 2012 May 4.

Mostafa GA, Al-Ayadhi LY. "Reduced serum concentrations of 25-hydroxy vitamin D in children with autism: Relation to autoimmunity." *J Neuroinflammation*. 2012 Aug 17;9:201.

Mowry EM, Waubant E, McCulloch CE, Okuda DT, Evangelista AA, Lincoln RR, Gourrand PA, Brenneman D, Owen MC, Qualley P, Bucci M, Hauser SL, Pelletier D. "Vitamin D status predicts new brain magnetic resonance imaging activity in multiple sclerosis." *Ann Neurol*. 2012 Aug;72(2):234-40.

Mulligan GB, Licata A. "Taking vitamin D with the largest meal improves absorption and results in higher serum levels of 25-hydroxyvitamin D." *J Bone Miner Res*. 2010 Apr;25(4):928-30.

Munger KL, Levin LI, Hollis BW, Howard NS, Asherio A. "Serum 25-hydroxyvitamin D levels and risk of multiple sclerosis." *JAMA*. 2006 Dec 20;296(23):2832-8.

Munger KL, Zhang SM, O'Reilly E, Hernan MA, Olek MJ, Willett WC, Asherio A. "Vitamin D intake and incidence of multiple sclerosis." *Neurology*. 2004 Jan 13;62(1):60-5.

Murray Michael T. *What the Drug Companies Won't Tell You and Your Doctor Doesn't Know*. Atria Books. 2009.

Neuhouser ML, Sorenson B, Hollis BW, Ambs A., Ulrich CM, McTiernan A, Berstein L, Gilliland F, Baumgartner R, Ballard-Barbash R. "Vitamin D insufficiency in a multiethnic cohort of breast cancer survivors." *Am J Clin Nutr*. 2008 Jul;88(1):133-9.

Nieves J, Cosman F, Herbert J, Shen V, Lindsay R. "High prevalence of vitamin D deficiency and reduced bone mass in multiple sclerosis." *Neurology*. 1994 Sep;44(9):1687-92.

Women with breast cancer have low vitamin D levels. *Women's Health Weekly* via NewsRx.com. October 23, 2009.

Oh EY, Ansell C, Nawaz H, Yang CH, Wood PA, Hrushesky WJ. "Global breast cancer seasonality." *Breast Cancer Res Treat.* 2010 Aug;123(1):233-243. Epub 2010 Feb 4.

Peppone LJ, Huston AJ, Reid ME, Rosier RN, Zakharia Y, Trump DL, Mustian KM, Janelsins MC, Purnell JQ, Morrow GR. "The effect of various vitamin D supplementation regimens in breast cancer patients." *Breast Cancer Res Treat.* 2011 May;127(1):171-7. Epub 2011 Mar 8.

Ramagopalan SV, Heger A, Berlanga AJ, Maugeri NJ, Lincoln MR, Burrell A, Handunnetthi L, Handel AE, Disanto G, Orton SM, Watson CT, Morahan JM, Giovannoni G, Ponting CP, Ebers GC, Knight JC. "A ChIP-seq defined genome-wide map of vitamin D receptor binding: associations with disease and evolution." *Genome Res.* 2010 Oct;20(10):1352-60. Epub 2010 Aug 24.

Ramagopalan SV, Maugeri NJ, Handunnetthi L, Lincoln MR, Orton, S-M, Dyment DA, DeLuca GC, Herrera BM, Chao MJ, Sadovnick AD, Ebers GC, Knight JC. "Expression of the multiple sclerosis-associated MHC Class II Allele HLA-DRB1*1501 is regulated by vitamin D." *PLoS Genet.* 2009 Feb;5(2): e1000369.

Reis JP, von Muehlen D, Miller ER 3rd, Michos ED, Appel LJ. "Vitamin D status and cardiometabolic risk factors in the United States adolescent population." *Pediatrics.* 2009 Sep;124(3):e371-9. Epub 2009 Aug 3.

Rheaume-Bleue, Kate. *Vitamin K₂ and the Calcium Paradox.* Wiley. 2012.

Rheem DS, Baylink DJ, Olafsson S, Jackson CS, Walter MH. "Prevention of colorectal cancer with vitamin D." *Scand J Gastroenterol.* 2010 Aug;45(7-8):775-84.

Richards JB, Valdes AM, Gardner JP, Paximadas D, Kimura M, Nessa A, Lu X, Surdulescu GL, Swaminathan R, Spector TD, Aviv A. "Higher serum vitamin D concentrations are associated with longer leukocyte telomere length in women." *Am J Clin Nutr.* 2007 Nov;86(5):1420-5.

Schwartz GG, Hulka BS. "Is vitamin D deficiency a risk factor for cancer? (Hypothesis)" *Anticancer Res.* 1990 Sep-Oct;10(5A):1307-11.

Scragg R. "Seasonality of cardiovascular disease mortality and the possible protective effect of ultraviolet radiation." *Int J Epidemiol.* 1981 Dec;10(4):337-41.

Shao T, Klein P, Grossbard ML. "Vitamin D and breast cancer." *Oncologist.* 2012;17(1):36-45. Epub 2012 Jan 10.

Tamer G, Arik S, Tamer I, Coksert D. "Relative vitamin D insufficiency in Hashimoto's thyroiditis." *Thyroid.* 2011 Aug;21(8):891-6. Epub 2011 Jul 13.

Trang HM, Cole DE, Rubin LA, Pierratos A, Siu S, Vieth, R. "Evidence that vitamin D_3 increases serum-25-hydroxyvitamin D more efficiently than does vitamin D_2." *Am J Clin Nutr.* 1998 Oct;68(4):854-8.

Tretli S, Schwartz GG, Torjesen PA, Robsahm TE. "Serum levels of 25-hydroxyvitamin D and survival in Norwegian patients with cancer of breast, colon, lung, and lymphoma: a population-based study." *Cancer Causes Control.* 2012 Feb;23(2):363-70. Epub 2011 Dec 23.

Tripkovic L, Lambert H, Hart K, Smith CP, Bucca G, Penson S, Chope G, Hypponen E, Berry J, Vieth R, Lanham-New S. "Comparison of vitamin D_2 and vitamin D_3 supplementation in raising serum 25-hydroxyvitamin D status: a systematic review and meta-analysis." *Am J Clin Nutr.* 2012 Jun;95(6):1357-64. Epub 2012 May 2.

Urashima M, Segawa T, Okazaki M, Kurihana M, Wada Y, Ida H. "Radomized trial of vitamin D supplementation to prevent seasonal influenza A in schoolchildren." *Am J Clin Nutr.* 2010 May;91(5):1255-60. Epub 2010 Mar 10.

VanAmerongen, BM, Dijkstra CD, Lips P, Polman CH. "Multiple sclerosis and vitamin D: an update." *Eur J Clin Nutr.* 2004 Aug;58(8):1095-109.

Varsavsky M, Reyes-Gracia R, Cortes-Berdonces N, Garcia-Martin A, Rozas-Moreno P, Munoz-Torres M. "Serum 25 OH vitamin D concentrations and calcium intake are low in patients with prostate cancer." *Endocrinol Nutr.* 2011 Nov;58(9):487-91. Epub 2011 Oct 20.

Viera VM, Hart JE, Webster TF, Weinberg J, Puett R, Laden F, Costenbader, KH, Karlson EW. "Association between residences in U.S. northern latitudes and rheumatoid arthritis: A spatial analysis of the Nurses' Health Study." *Environ Health Perspect.* 2010 Jul;118(7):957-61. Epub 2010 Mar 25.

Vieth R. "Vitamin D supplementation, 25-hydroxyvitamin D concentrations, and safety." *Am J Clin Nutr.* 1999;69(5):842-56.

Walker, Richard W., Jr. *African-American Healthy.* Square One Publishers. 2011.

Ward KA, Das G, Berry JL, Roberts SA, Rawer R, Adams JE, Mughal Z. "Vitamin D status and muscle function in post-menarchal adolescent girls." *J Clin Endocrinol Metab.* 2009 February; 94(2):559-63.

Wei MY, Garland CF, Gorham ED, Mohr SB, Giovannucci E. "Vitamin D and prevention of colorectal adenoma: a meta-analysis." *Cancer Epidemol Biomarkers Prev.* 2008 Nov;17(11):2958-69.

Wortsman J, Matsuoka LY, Chen TC, Lu Z, Holick MF. "Decreased bioavailability of vitamin D in obesity." Am J Clin Nutr. 2000 Sep;72(3):690-3. Erratum in: *Am J Clin Nutr.* 2003 May;77(5):1342.

Yamashita H, Noguchi S, Takatsu K, Koike E, Murakami T, Watanabe S, Uchino S, Yamashita H, Kawamoto H. "High prevalence of vitamin D deficiency in Japanese female patients with Graves' disease." *Endocr J.* 2001 Feb;48(1):63-9.

Zaidi, Sarfraz. *Power of Vitamin D.* Outskirts Press, Inc. 2010.

About the Author

Susan "Sue" Rex Ryan was born and raised in the Philadelphia, Pennsylvania area. She earned a bachelor of science degree at Georgetown University, concentrating on languages and linguistics. Sue also holds a master of science degree from the National War College in Washington, D.C.

In her early fifties, Sue was surprised to learn that her quality of life was not what she had expected due to declining health. She realized that her medical issues were primarily a result of hormonal imbalances. Inspired by a Suzanne Somers' seminar on pursuing natural solutions to health issues, Sue embarked on an incredible health journey by exploring natural approaches to improve her health. She also conducted extensive medical research and attended medical conferences and seminars where she earned Continuing Medical Education credits. Her professional memberships include the Vitamin D Council and the American Academy of Anti-Aging Medicine.

Defend Your Life is Sue's first book. Her sincere wish is that everyone—men and women of all ages and backgrounds—improves their quality of life by safely, inexpensively, and easily taking an effective vitamin D_3 supplement. Since attaining adequate vitamin D_3 levels, Sue's quality of life significantly has improved. She hopes that your life as well the lives of your loved ones and friends will benefit from this wonderful nutrient.

Sue and her husband Dave reside in the sunny suburbs of beautiful Las Vegas, Nevada. They enjoy traveling to visit family and friends, as well as experiencing life in far-flung locations including Easter Island and French Polynesia.

Visit www.vitaminD3book.com for more vitamin D_3 information. Drop by www.SusanRexRyan.com and follow Sue's commentary on Twitter @VitD3Sue.

SOUTHBOROUGH LIBRARY

CPSIA information can be obtained at www.ICGtesting.com
Printed in the USA
LVOW121538150513

333966LV00019B/802/P